# Tinnitus

LESLIE SHEPPARD & AUDREY HAWKRIDGE

# Tinnitus

*Learning to live with it*

ASHGROVE PRESS, BATH

First published in Great Britain by
ASHGROVE PRESS LIMITED
4 Brassmill Centre, Brassmill Lane
Bath BA1 3JN

and distributed in the USA by
Avery Publishing Group Inc.
350 Thorens Avenue
Garden City Park
New York 11040

First published 1987
Second printing 1989

British Library Cataloguing in Publication Data

Sheppard, Leslie
    Tinnitus: learning to live with it.
    1. Tinnitus
    I. Title   II. Hawkridge, Audrey
    617.8      RF293.8
            ISBN 0-906798-80-9 Pbk

Photoset in 10½/12pt Palatino by
Ann Buchan (Typesetters), Middlesex
Printed and bound by
Hillman Printers (Frome) Ltd, Frome, Somerset

# Contents

# Preface

This book gives an excellent interpretation of the overall sociological effects produced by tinnitus. The authors' own suffering is highlighted in an empathetic way and it would make good supportive reading, especially for the new tinnitus sufferer.

The British Tinnitus Association is indebted to Leslie Sheppard in acclaiming our work by contributing 50% of his royalties to tinnitus research. This book would be on a B.T.A. recommended reading list.

DAVID WIGGINS, CO-ORDINATOR
BRITISH TINNITUS ASSOCIATION

# PART I

# Sounds Nasty

A Personal Account by

AUDREY HAWKRIDGE

*With loving thanks*
     *to John*
*for sharing the tinnitus with me*
     *and Ian*
*for improvising my emergency 'masker'*
     *and discovering the BTA*


                              *Audrey Hawkridge*

# Acknowledgements

My grateful acknowledgements to Mr Jonathan Hazell for his helpful advice, and the British Tinnitus Association for their kind permission to quote from newsletters.

# Sounds Nasty

This is the story of a 'tinnitus case': unwilling entrant to an ever-expanding club. It isn't a new club, in fact it's at least a couple of thousand years old, but today membership is increasing dramatically. There are more of us around, of course, and we are subjected to the stresses and viruses of the modern world, as well as to a different, measurable kind of assault: sound, from mechanical and electronic devices which are the background to most of our work and play. Who knows how much of all this contributes towards those more insidious sounds, surplus to requirements and gloomy evidence of the body's treachery to the soul, the sounds of tinnitus?

No two people seem to suffer from what the ancient Greeks called 'noises from within' in exactly the same way. This is a very private form of distress, unfortunately, as you just can't get under someone else's skin, or inside someone else's ears! So the only experience I can really write about is my own. But as it carries in the end a message of hope (unlike most messages you are given on the subject) perhaps it will help a little if I share that experience with you.

Elsewhere in this book you will find where to look for assistance, and what is generally known about causes and therapy. This is mainly just a personal record of coming to terms with a miserable condition which a few years ago hardly anyone ever spoke of, yet which, it now transpires, blights several million people's lives the world over. Cut off in frightening isolation, unnoticed because outsiders can't detect that there's anything wrong, and a long way down bureaucracy's 'urgent research' list, these millions seem condemned for a long time ahead to suffer in silence.

Well, not exactly silence. . . .

* * *

*Tinnitus*

1

At around 11 p.m. on June 24th 1980 I laid my head on my pillow and went off to sleep amid the beloved, boring old still of the night – for the last time.

I had no idea it was going to be a momentous occasion; no inner voice warned me to savour it like the historic pre-execution breakfast. Yet momentous it was, for when I sat up in bed the next morning, the buzzing of the alarm clock was accompanied by another far more devastating noise in my right ear: a thick, elephantine vacuum cleaner hoovering its relentless way over the untrodden carpets of my brain.

I shook my head, hit my ear, swallowed hard, and went through all the rites (except gum-chewing, unthinkable at 6.30 a.m.), which helpful airline staff used to suggest in order to combat ear problems, in the far-off days before pressurised jet travel was invented. But the vacuum cleaner persisted – joined, to my horror, about half an hour later by a piercing whistle in the left ear.

'A bit of catarrh,' the family murmured comfortingly at various stages during the day. 'You're probably in for a cold.'

Well, I thought, in a lifetime of catching colds, I've never had one that started this way. However, change of some sort was obviously imminent, for the cleaner finished its work by the evening of the 26th, and altered to a heavy shushing hiss, while the steady whistle in the other ear still provided a monotonous, unmusical and painfully shrill descant. At times the timpani came in too, with a muted thunder of glugs and gurgles, like bathwater pouring down a pipe to the sound of wildly unrhythmic drumbeats. This was really something else. Tactile, almost. Disturbing too, for the pressure was downright explosive when I went back to that less peaceful pillow at night. And it came from within pushing outwards, instead of the more acceptable direction for pressure to take, from outside pushing in.

Still, there was always the chance that it *was* a cold, or something similar. My digestive system chose to misbehave that week (and for many subsequent weeks too) and I had a sore throat with uncomfortable neck glands, plus intermittent dizziness. So, cheered rather than disheartened by this motley collection of symptoms, I resigned myself patiently to waiting for it to run its course.

Two months went by. I gave up the patient waiting and visited the group surgery on the outskirts of the large provincial city where I then lived. Not for the shushing and whistling – still with me, to my surprise – but for the one other remaining annoyance, which seemed more urgent because it was extremely uncomfortable, cramping to my social style, and costing me a fortune on the famous mixture of an Eminent Crimean War Physician.

Having usually found that if you try and press someone for two things at once you get neither, I said nothing about the noises. Anyway, one doesn't wish to appear a hypochondriac in front of a stranger; and my own doctor was away on holiday. One of his partners dealt with me kindly – blood test, hospital appointment and all – upon which my alimentary system immediately took the law into its own perverse hands and calmed down unaided.

Nearly three more months passed. The bright days of June had now given place to murky November. Apart from slight dizziness at times, everything was back to normal. Except for the noises, going strong as always. Very strong. They had changed now to a more strident sound, the same in both ears, (or, morbid thought, did they start from further inside still?), and far from showing the improvement I'd been sure must ultimately come, they were getting worse.

At this point I tried some home-spun remedies, inhaling Menthol and Eucalyptus and Friar's Balsam until my eyes streamed, and pumping Waxol in from the opposite direction until my ears were so full of liquid that the Sounds were the only things I could hear. But nothing worked. It was obviously neither catarrh nor wax. Some little bug that would respond to anti-biotics, perhaps? In my innocence I decided I'd waited long enough; it was high time that the professionals came onto the scene and got rid of the problem once and for all.

Back to the surgery. It seemed wiser to keep with the same man as before, so I did. But that was a mistake. Highly respected and conscientious doctor though he had a reputation for being, he was so out of his element on the strange ground of tinnitus that he underwent an astonishing personality change.

Let it be said here and now that I have the greatest respect for G.P.s on the whole. I have close friends in the profession, and I go to an excellent doctor at present, as well as having found many an excellent doctor in the past. How they manage to do their comprehensive jobs and still keep up with new developments is a mystery to me, and a source of admiration. But one can be unlucky, even so. Particularly tinnitus sufferers, perhaps, for ours is a Cinderella condition. Since it is rarely dangerous – except to sanity in extreme cases, and thereby maybe to life – and since it is something they can't see, many doctors do apparently treat its victims with stony indifference.

Blissfully ignorant of this as yet, I looked him squarely in the eye, (to convince him that I was not an over-imaginative neurotic doing a latter-day Joan of Arc act), and began my tale of woe. Hyperbole was very tempting, but I avoided it and stuck firmly to succinct fact. However, I needn't have bothered about the small matter of presentation, for just as I was getting into my stride, I saw a glazed look come over his face.

'Just a minute,' he said, turning away from me. He then picked up the internal telephone to his receptionist and proceeded to transmit a message about something totally unconnected with my dreary little case, which hadn't taken up enough of his attention to stop his mind from wandering. There's no way of measuring the urgency of other people's phone calls, of course; maybe this one was a matter of life and death, but I can only state that it sounded unhurried. At length he turned to me again, replacing the receiver. 'Sorry about that,' he mumbled. 'Now, you were saying. . . .?'

Crushing though the weight of his boredom was, I repeated my spiel. But instead of falling off to sleep as I'd feared, he was suddenly galvanised into action.

'Stand up!' he barked. Startled, I leapt to attention, at which he poked a light briskly down each ear. 'Any dizziness?' he asked.

'Well, I have had, a little,' I answered.

He sat down and leaned back in his chair with an air of

satisfied finality. 'You have,' he announced, 'a condition known as Ménière's Syndrome.'

I fought back the urge to ask why, if that were so, I didn't feel sick, and why the noise was so much worse than the dizziness. For, after all, he had given the matter at least one and a half seconds' deliberation, so who was I to question his diagnosis? He scribbled a prescription for some tablets, smiled me out of the doorway and with a cheery shrug delivered the parting shot – that if they didn't work I should have to 'learn to live with the noise.' That very phrase. The one trotted out to all tinnitus sufferers. Only I didn't know that then; it almost sounded like an original thought straight from the heart.

To his credit, however, he did not abandon me then and there. He made a further appointment for several weeks ahead, and when I returned to report no change, he gave me another lot of the same tablets. A few days later all hell exploded.

* * *

## 2

I would not have believed it possible for the human body to produce the volume of spontaneous sound which attacked me from then on. It stabbed in long throbbing crescendoes to an unbearable screech like that of an old-fashioned railway engine letting off steam at close quarters. Every so often it would tantalise me, almost more unbearably, by shutting off altogether, and giving me a split second or two of the golden silence I had never appreciated before. Then it would rise again, thin, thickening, then screaming in successive surges, to stay at top strength for hours or sometimes days at a stretch. My whole brain, my whole life in fact, was condensed into one great shrieking whistle that shut off at source all power of thought, all desire for communication, all interest in the outside world, all confidence, all humour, and every shred of capacity for pleasure. I was trapped – imprisoned inside a tight dense claustrophobic bubble of ear-splitting sound. On the rare occasions I could get outside myself and be objective, the whole situation seemed like pure science fiction.

At this stage life grew very black indeed. Before long, and without knowing the complexities of inner ear structure, I wondered quite seriously if I could persuade any surgeon to destroy my hearing altogether. To be stone deaf would be infinitely preferable to this fiendish bombardment. Luckily for me, I didn't know at the time that such an operation would be the height of madness, since it could make the tinnitus even louder; so for a little while it was a comfort to think that there might be this last-ditch possibility available.

Worse still, and difficult though I now find this to believe on looking back, I know that ideas of suicide hovered, and sometimes lingered, in my mind. They never actually settled, mainly because I had one incomparable blessing, a cheerfully sympathetic husband who came home to me each night, and put aside his own tiredness at the end of a long and hard day's work by talking to me about anything and everything he could think of to stir up my dulled wits and flagging spirits. Quiet cheerfulness and sympathy in the right balance – a lot of the first and not *too* much of the second – are, in fact, the most valuable crumbs of comfort a partner can offer. The sad thing about tinnitus is that it usually strikes in middle age, when one is likely to be living alone, perhaps for the first time, and the sufferer has to search outside home for the right companionship to lift the burden.

Recognising that I was therefore in a better plight than many people similarly smitten – if there were indeed any others out there, for I'd not heard of them so far – I tried to think positively, an expression which was very popular at the time, and which now appeared to be tailor-made for my requirements.

First, medication. Needless to say, I stopped taking the tablets. Marvellous though they might be for most Ménière's cases, they clearly weren't the cure for me. (Because, it later turned out, I wasn't a Ménière's case at all!)

Was there in fact ever going to be a cure? Or even easement? Apparently not. By this time I'd scoured every library shelf for miles around, and the miniscule amount of reading matter on the subject was unremittingly depressing. Every little treatise on tinnitus repeated the doctor's dictum: you have to learn to live with it. Well, up to a point I suppose there is truth in that. But what they didn't tell me was that things don't always stay the same. The tinnitus itself can diminish very, very gradually over a period of years. Like watching the hour hand of a clock, it is so slow that you aren't aware it's happening until you look back. Or the brain may accept the noise – as an E.N.T. consultant was to tell me a year hence – to such a degree that it can actually switch it off at times just prior to sleep and at first awakening, so that you could swear for a moment it had gone away. Until of course on properly waking up it comes back with such a violent din as to prove how overworked the poor old brain must have been, plugging the metaphorical dyke with its finger all night long! However, I must confess that in these dreadful earlier days I was not so fortunate as to have my nights blessed by this built-in shut-off system. My brain was still stunned by the new and fearsome beating it was taking, and hadn't yet got round to combating it. Which brings me to positive thinking again:-

Second, the problem of bedtime. The mind – as a conscious, spiritual organ – strives to adjust, even while the brain – a more mechanical piece of equipment – is still reeling. And amid all its inner weeping, resentment and fear, it has to face going to bed every night with as much equanimity as it can muster up. For me, the bathwater with drum accompaniment continued to provide its unorthodox and painful lullaby, only made bearable by the effort of trying to turn it into a sort of pattern, which, as it didn't branch out into too much variation, was almost calming in its horrible predictability. But it was louder these days than it had been at first. And it would shift in volume to whichever side was away from the pillow. The usual nocturnal programme worked to a rota, each with its own tribulations:

1 Turn on right side, put up with thumping till left ear bursts.
2 Turn on left side, put up with thumping till right ear bursts.
3 Turn on back, and listen to thumping coming from everywhere, as well of course as that permanent piercing hell-whistle.

Then (1) again, and so on. Ears don't actually burst, I know, but they can feel pretty close to it.

Eventually exhaustion brings sleep, but at that time the noises often woke me up again, thus confounding a theory I toyed with, that it was all in the mind and didn't happen when I wasn't sitting waiting for it.

While on the subject of sleep, don't drop off during the daytime! Easier said than done, but sometimes a snooze in the armchair can be staved off by a mighty effort at the eleventh hour, and the dog can have an extra walk instead, maybe. I have found, ever since the first onset of tinnitus, that the horrendous upsurge of sound which assaults me on waking from a short nap is a thousand times worse than the increase following a night's sleep. Even a moment's nodding-off can produce it. I soon learned that if I felt sleepy during the day it was worth struggling to do something energetic to keep the horror at bay; and this is not just my experience, but a fairly general one. In fact, the more energetic I became in those bad old days, the quieter the noises. Positive thinking again. . .

Third, keep active. Mentally as well as physically, in whatever ratio your preferences lie. A brisk walk in the cold air of that first winter – if possible carrying a load of shopping to make the effort greater! – could thin out the sound to a rather more acceptable level, lasting for anything up to half an hour. Not much of a bonus, maybe, but better than nothing. And on one bitter February weekend away in Cambridge, a walk round King's College Chapel and gardens in freezing wind reduced the sound to a thin, high reedy whistle which was perfect bliss by comparison with my normal railway-engine-letting-off-steam volume. And the effect of that lasted all the evening.

Chewing over these weird phenomena with my husband, whose medical knowledge is about on a par with mine (at a 'pop' level) but who looks for the practical solution to all aspects of the unknown, he offered the theory that adrenalin had something to do with it. And he was possibly right, for recent thinking appears to indicate that adrenalin flow has some bearing on tinnitus.

Actual and physical results apart, bodily exercise – if you

normally enjoy it – can be beneficial simply because it gives you something to concentrate on. The harder and more complicated the task, the more you can dismiss the tinnitus, so that perhaps a game of tennis might have more value than a jog along the beach. But *do* something, if you can. Or, alternatively, *think* hard about something.

My own special hobby is history, in a lot of shapes and forms. I'd already produced several little historical offerings, which had met with roughly the same kind of reception from publishers as my tinnitus met with in the doctor's surgery. But one can't afford to be daunted by a few cold shoulders, so I thrashed about frantically for some hard work to concentrate on as an aid to sanity, something which would take up all my attention and distract me from the infernal racket going on inside my head. No one had so far ever translated the love-letters of one of the most fascinating figures of French history, Henri IV, so it struck me that if I could put them into English, it could be an undertaking with maybe even some material profit at the end of it. (It wasn't, but that hardly mattered. And it had been rather a forlorn hope in the middle of a recession!) From then on, in a side room of my local library, with a poignant – to me – appeal for silence on its wall, I tussled with 120 letters in Old French, and triumphantly put them into updated English with explanatory trimmings.

At this point my husband departed momentarily from his role of supporter-in-chief. Happening to glance by accident at a couple, he expressed the opinion that if he couldn't have written better love-letters than those, he'd have 'phoned instead – a view presumably shared by the one or two editors who overcame commercial misgivings and agreed to have a preliminary look. Well, they didn't see the spiciest ones; I hadn't done them then. . .

Anyway, the work served its purpose. For one thing, it had enlightened me as to the writer's character. Covering a large span of his life as they did, the letters represented three facets of this perennial royal lover, chopped up into well-defined compartments of soldier, romantic, and proverbial 'old fool.' Even if nobody else found that interesting, I did. And that was what counted.

Far more important, I'd achieved my object. I'd found the

work totally absorbing, if difficult; and it didn't matter how little it grabbed anyone else, so long as it had kept me occupied. (That is the point, really. Let the world think what it may of your own particular brand of therapy, so long as it suits you.) I had used those first terrible months to good effect, proving I could still get down to problems which were quite gruelling at times, my French being appallingly rusty. And I could do it under ceaseless aural stress – getting away from the noise rather than staying shut in with it. And that was the secret of how to fight it, I felt. It would never be as bad again, now I knew that secret.

I shall always be grateful to Henri IV and his three chief mistresses. They saw me through a very bad patch, and helped me ride it out successfully. Everyone has his or her own panacea, not usually as bizarre as mine. Mentally or physically, whatever you work really hard at, and extend yourself over, will keep your attention away from your distress. I am making heavy weather of this point because for much of the time advice on the subject seems to be to the contrary. One is often told to rest, to stay quiet and relaxed and to try not to tire oneself. For me that has been proved wrong. The worst thing I could do was to sit and rest. Mentally it encouraged introspection, and physically it merely created more noise.

\* \* \*

### 3

During this period, abandoning all thought of further medical help, I'd virtually discharged myself from the doctor's care, by going back when the next six-weekly appointment was due and saying that I didn't think his tablets did a lot for me, but I was finding it all easier to come to terms with anyhow. We parted with mutual relief and bright smiles all round, and I returned home to try and work things out some other way.

I began to discover that all sorts of mechanical and electrical devices had interesting effects, either beneficial or the reverse. Crowd noise on television was dreadful, producing a condition known in tinnitus circles as 'recruitment,' (i.e. it recruits further reserves of noise to come to the aid of those which are already engaged in battle against you). Snooker was therefore much better to watch than football! Television itself causes trouble to many people; irrespective of the sound you can actually hear on it, it apparently transmits a virtually unheard note which can be aggravating. On the other hand, its value as a distracting agent may counterbalance this particular evil. Also, freezers or fridge-freezers are troublesome to some people. I have had a rather noisy one for the last ten years, which probably didn't help in the initial stages; yet now I'm no more bothered by it than anyone else would be.

A mixed blessing, or curse, may be your car engine. Some worked well for me on long journeys; others were torture even on short ones. So I couldn't come to any conclusions at all on that score. But a study of the good things came up with some unexpected results. Some of the best sounds I found for temporary easing of the problem at that time were the clatter of an old-fashioned typewriter, the telephone, the vacuum cleaner, and 'white noise' on radio – the benefit from these lasting up to five minutes. Hardly worth bothering about? On the contrary: salvation. Not just for the little bit of peace, but for the little bit of hope, warranted or otherwise.

Having finished those old royal love-letters, I decided to have a go at a novel, and bonked away on my ancient typewriter for an hour or so every day – noticing with delight that after typing only a page, perhaps, I would get two or three minutes' respite of silence. This of course led to a strange work-schedule, with lots of short spurts and short rests, slowing the production line down a bit but providing a touch of relief at intervals. The telephone was a wonderful quietener of a different sort. A very brief conversation didn't do anything, but a longish one gave, again, two or three minutes' peace afterwards. Apart from conversations – which can get out of hand and turn into a financial nightmare – I could always dial a bedtime story, and did so more than once to good effect. As for the vacuum cleaner, the benefit of that lasted slightly longer, a good five minutes. Need I say that we had cleaner carpets than ever before or since? Last but not least of the four, the radio white noise. This was not my idea, but it proved a winner.

We have two grown-up sons. One lived at the time in America, and so was obviously not in a position to give support. The other was London-based, and we exchanged visits every so often. On one of these visits he donated a pair of his earphones to me. Plugging them in to our portable radio, he tuned it to a short wave off-station rushing sound which once upon a time I'd have flinched from with a shudder.

'White noise could be what you need,' he said. 'Try it for a bit and see if it helps.' To my great joy it did. So from then on, whenever the whistling became too terrible to stand with fortitude, I would sit sheltered within those earphones and listen thankfully to static – the volume variable to order, and under my instant control. (Six years later, I now look back on that as one of my lifelines; but the situation is so much better these days that several months ago I gave him back his earphones).

This improvised substitute for a masker was to serve very effectively for quite a long time, usually used in about ten-minute bursts. And while it might not suit everyone, it was better for my purposes, I felt, than an orthodox masker of the kind generally recommended, which would have to be fitted like a hearing aid, and could be expensive, especially in my health authority area. I'd read a bit about maskers by then, and knew that they were not available to me under the National Health Service system, so as a consequence one would cost at least £200. Both of my ears were affected equally, so it seemed to me that masking in one alone would be more of an irritant than a relief, and masking in both might not only be a rather costly experiment but could create a shut-in feeling. So, I reasoned, if I did invest in one (or two) I'd want to switch it (them) off too frequently to make them worth trying.

Concerning maskers, mine is a minority view, I think. Many people swear by them, and a trial is recommended by all those involved in tinnitus treatment. The typical masking sound is of flowing water or waves on the seashore – temperamentally pleasing as well as a soothing contrast to the cacophony within. I survived my worst time without normal masking, and mercifully don't feel the need for it now. But, as

I said, things don't stay the same. And if one day in the future I'm reduced to considering maskers, it's good to know they do help other people and actually can improve hearing, it seems.

But, to return to my accidental discoveries in the field of sound helping sound, the prize-winner in these stakes was the London Underground. On my rare trips to London, I used to enjoy spending a few hours in the British Museum, where I had a reader's ticket to the British Library. I use the word 'enjoy' advisedly, for in a muted way enjoyment was beginning by this stage to come back, here and there. And it was on the first of these post-tinnitus-onset excursions, after a forty minute ride on the Central Line from the suburb where I was staying, that I suddenly realised the statutory silence of the Reading Room was, in truth, silence! I couldn't believe it. I shuffled my books around, just to make certain I hadn't gone totally deaf, and was reassured. Throughout my whole sojourn there that day, concentration was ironically well below par, because I kept getting carried away with ecstatic ideas of permanent freedom from noise once more, and had to control a ridiculous urge to get up and do a victory dance all round the hallowed circle of tome-filled shelves. Incredibly, that silence lasted till evening, the first real break I'd had, and the brightly-lit signpost to better things in the future.

Nothing else, unfortunately, was able to manufacture such magic. And unless you have to commute to work by this method, it's impractical as well as cripplingly expensive to spend too many hours a day on the Tube! Perhaps it wouldn't be right for other people, in any case. As I've said before, no two sufferers are exactly alike in their experiences. But I present it as a possible means of alleviation, for what it's worth. It did the trick for me every time, and on one or two occasions the full flood of nasty sound didn't return until the following morning – an unprecedented bonanza.

Nowadays I find my sound patterns are for the most part quieter, steadier and less affected by outside influences, except for that background noise of perpetually shouting crowds on television: still troublesome. But during the years between, when the tinnitus was dying down – so slowly as to be imperceptible – I found the old 'cures' could change into bugbears, or just stop being useful. While telephoning and

carpet cleaning gradually ceased to make any difference one
way or another, typing changed from friend to foe, and made
matters worse. So it really is a case of discovering what is right
for you, and always being prepared for it to turn wrong
overnight!

* * *

4

About a year after I was first smitten, I thought I'd have
another try at seeing what the medical profession could do for
me. While the most intense horrors had subsided a fraction,
things had stayed pretty bad for much of the time. I still vaguely
thought of myself as having Ménière's Disease, though by
now the dizziness had long gone – to be replaced later by a
weird vision-on-sound sensation, with four oscillations to
the heartbeat, visible whether my eyes were open or shut;
this luckily only assaulted me at times when the sound was
really bad. In any event, it seemed silly not to seek the help of a
consultant. I went to my own doctor – not the one whom I'd
seen before – and explained the position. He sent me to a
consultant attached to the big hospital in the city nearby, and
I was put through some exhaustive and sophisticated tests.

He was a very pleasant and thorough man, who investigated that original Ménière's diagnosis as a start. I was
strapped to a movable couch and turned over from side to
side. I had hot and cold water alternately shot into my ears and
the time taken to adjust from the ensuing giddiness
measured. I was put in a small dark room with sensors stuck
all over my head, and something else was measured there –
I'm not sure what. And (quite pleasant by contrast) I was
made to walk a straight line without looking. At the end of all
these trials by ordeal, I was pronounced not guilty. Sorry, I
mean not afflicted. It wasn't Ménière's Disease.

So what was it? A virus, he thought. Would it ever get
better? Well, no, unfortunately. But, he said, I would grow to
notice it less; he could almost promise that. (It was then that
he described the brain's peculiar pre-sleeping and post-

waking tricks I've mentioned before.) He didn't actually say in as many words that I should 'have to learn to live with it,' but the gist of his speech undoubtedly leaned that way. However, he said, there was one remedy which might just work, not as a complete cure, but possibly it could improve matters a bit. Accordingly he prescribed for me some tablets normally used to help along blood circulation. He explained that in some cases tinnitus can be made a little easier by an extra boost of circulation to inner ear cells affected by otherwise irreversible virus damage. After taking them for a month I was to go back to him and report progress.

During that month I felt as if I could have moved mountains. Galloping up stairs which usually seemed steep, and racing around as if I had a runaway engine inside me, the feeling of general wellbeing – accompanied, however, by some slightly unnerving inner pumpings! – was quite unique. And it did certainly seem that the noise thinned out a tiny bit. However, I was conservative in my comments on this when I returned to him, because there were already patches of slightly thinner and quieter tinnitus by now anyway. Few and far between, but they existed, making minor improvements difficult to assess.

I mentioned the strange sensation of being a sort of potential Wonder Woman. He replied that he might have expected me to say I had indigestion, perhaps, but not really anything else. Alas, he was telling me about indigestion too late, for the seeds were already sown. Soon after I went home clutching my next batch of tablets, my hypersensitive system went into action. . . But that's another story, too boring to go into here.

My verdict, overall, on his treatment was that it did probably do a little bit of good; the sounds were never quite so thick again, at least not on a regular basis. But I don't really think that the gradual and slow improvement over the years was connected with that at all. And I couldn't help wishing, seeing the trouble it caused me, that either the consultant who prescribed the tablets or the doctor who did his bidding had told me the drawbacks in advance. I understand their reasons; they are asked to cure one condition, and one alone. In the case of consultants that is naturally the only aspect they are looking at, anyway, and it may often be connected with research which is important to them. If they worried about side-effects in occasional cases they'd get nowhere. But it would be nice to have the power of choosing, yourself, whether you should take a chance on something that might not agree with one part of you, for the sake of possible benefit to another part. You wouldn't expect to buy any other kind of commodity without being given an opportunity to decide if the price was too high, would you?

One more thing before I leave the subject of doctors. Again, I appreciate their difficulties, dealing as I'm sure they do with many an imaginary invalid sprinkled among their genuine cases. But it amazed me that even with my most graphic descriptions of the noise I was subjected to, none of them even began to comprehend the swamping volume of it all.

My own doctor, experienced and wise though he was, had responded to my tale of night-time misery with the remark that of course everything sounded louder at night anyway. And the consultant, on my third and last visit, had followed up a depressing prediction that within a year I might need a hearing aid, (fortunately incorrect), with a question which really astounded me. He actually asked if, now I had said the tinnitus was marginally better, I could still hear it against our conversation.

I laughed, hollowly. I think I must have gaped at him too, for he looked a little surprised. But then I remembered that he was after all a sincere, kindly man who had no real and scientific means of knowing whether my complaining was justified or exaggerated. So I managed to remain quiet and polite.

'Yes, I can still hear the tinnitus through the conversation,' I said meekly. 'The only difference is that now I don't have to strain quite so hard to hear the conversation through the tinnitus.'

\* \* \*

## 5

To date I haven't had any more encounters with the medical

profession regarding tinnitus. I think most G.P.s understand it better now. Some water has gone under the bridge since then, and there has been a huge upsurge in general awareness. Much of this is due to a more open attitude to stress, and greater willingness to talk about it. When you have a stress-related condition these days, it is the done thing to describe it to saturation point, to anyone who will listen – whereas a few years ago you'd have been afraid of being dismissed as a neurotic who needed to pull yourself together, if you'd started talking to people about hearing noises in your head. And a few years earlier still, you'd have ranked as a lunatic, fit only for the nearest asylum!

Fear that their tinnitus was a sign of terminal illness, fear that they were going mad or would in any case be thought mad, even just fear of ridicule – all these have kept many a sufferer quiet in the past. Not so now. This is the Age of Discussion.

But, on a more precise scale, recent awareness of tinnitus can be a result of its case being taken up in public. Firstly, in Parliament, by the M.P. Jack Ashley, who has done so much for the deaf and who early in 1985 presented to the Commons a petition with 72,000 signatures pleading against the impending closure of the Tinnitus Clinic at University College Hospital, London. This clinic, run by Jonathan Hazell, Medical Research Fellow to the Royal National Institute for the Deaf, does valuable and varied work in the fields of both research and treatment, and its continuance was threatened for a while due to government spending cuts. Luckily, Mr Ashley (and perhaps the weight of the 72,000 signatures too) effected a stay of execution, it seems. At the time of writing no decision has been come to yet.

Secondly, the media has played its part in recent years. Naturally, media coverage always increases public knowledge a millionfold. And in 1984 Radio 4 broadcast an excellent half-hour award-winning talk on tinnitus, twice repeated I believe. This cannot have failed to create interest and contribute to understanding.

An earlier and shorter talk on the subject, broadcast one morning in 1981, was a great breakthrough for me. My thoughtful London son happened to hear it by chance, locked

onto it, and made a note of the name and address of an
organisation which neither G.P.s nor consultant had told me
about, but which has been the prop and saviour of so many
sufferers since it was first founded in 1979 – the British
Tinnitus Association.

BTA is under the wing of the Royal National Institute for
the Deaf, located at 105 Gower Street, London, WC1E 6AH.
The Association is open to anyone and only charges you what
you want to donate – and that's an easy price to pay for the
comfort it affords! It presides over research, gives addresses of
its locally based self-help groups, offers practical guidance
and information, and sends out a quarterly newsletter which
above all makes you realise you aren't alone. There are letters
in it written by people in all states of mind, ranging from
those who have conquered their distress, and those who are
striving to do so but haven't succeeded yet, to those who are
tragically beaten down by the sudden, unfair attack from an
enemy whose existence they had never envisaged in their
wildest nightmares. Whatever category of sufferer you
identify yourself with, you'll find somebody else there like
you; one glance through the letters to the editor tells every
lonely prisoner shut off behind a high wall of sound that there
are a lot of other people similarly imprisoned behind their
own high walls. Three hundred thousand or so severe cases in
Britain, at the last count.

And the known ones are only the tip of the iceberg. Ten of
my friends and acquaintances – totally unconnected with
BTA or any similar organisation – have tinnitus. And I know
of several others, through my social grapevine. As far as I can
tell, just one of them found his way, once, to a consultant's
rooms – where the only thing of note he was told was that he'd
soon go deaf. (It didn't happen!) So there is a vast unknown
army of people walking around with greater or lesser
buzzings, whistlings, thumpings, whinings, chirrupings,
shriekings, rushings, roarings, bell-ringings, hummings,
barkings, hissings, and all kinds of more harmonious sounds,
from single notes in a repeated progression to a full orchestra.

All that suffering, indiscernible to the outside world, except
perhaps for taut expressions and sleepless bags under the
eyes! Everybody used to say to me when the flow was in full

spate, 'You *look* perfectly all right!' Disbelief could tend to flicker over their faces, and the subject might be changed to one that lent itself more readily to bright two-way chat. There were exceptions; some people are naturally gifted at spotting trouble and striking a perfect balance between sympathy and sensible distraction, and some are trained for it by virtue of their careers. But the only person who could detect at a glance whether I was having a good day or a bad one was my husband. 'Fouler than usual?' he'd ask sometimes as he entered the door at night. One or twice he was wrong, but only if I had toothache or something instead.

\* \* \*

6

There's a timeworn music-hall joke which everyone knows:
  'I've got bells in my ears, so I went to the doctor.'
  'Did he do you any good?'
  'Yes, I can hear them much better now.'
  Hoary though this is, it's worth quoting here, because it does illustrate one type of attitude to tinnitus, displayed by the sort of person who'll go off into peals of happy laughter at other people's mild disasters. Banana-skin humour, really.
  A hairdresser I went to was like that. He was telling me a funny story about a party he'd been at, against the background of ear-splitting radio and a nearby blow-dryer. Afraid that I'd miss the punch-line, I shouted that I couldn't quite hear him with all these other noises going on, and mentioned my difficulty in one or two briefly bellowed words.
  'Oh, no!' he chortled, 'Got your own party going on inside your head, have you?' – and he proceeded to fall about with uncontrolled mirth. There's nothing you can do at times like that but smile wanly and look as if you're sharing the joke.
  When it was new and very preoccupying, I observed that my condition was treated by most other people with hesitant delicacy. Some shied away from talking about it at all. They would, I think, be the same people who might shy away from

speaking to the newly bereaved: those naturally reluctant to step on unfamiliar conversational ground, those afraid of saying the wrong thing, or those who feel they can't console in the face of an incurable condition.

In some ways this is a pity, if at rock bottom they would like to be helpful. For, like the newly bereaved, very few of the newly-stricken-with-tinnitus are themselves reluctant to talk, as a rule. On the contrary, they are more often than not cheered up by other people's interest and concern, and are often longing for the safety valve provided by a sympathetic ear – absolutely anybody's! And positive answers to the trouble aren't required, because the talker knows as well as the listener that there are none. Mere passive listening with an occasional understanding nod or comment can work wonders, particularly for the sufferer who lives alone.

I found out one amazing thing: people are loth to ask after your ears! Perhaps it's some aspect of deep-seated primaeval psychology. After all, ears are orifices, which makes them one of nature's less mentionable creations. And they're not always frightfully clean in their habits, either. Whatever the reason, everyone avoided the use of the word 'ears' in my first bad days. Sometimes they were put into the singular instead. To have one ear go rogue in such a ludicrous fashion was a matter of sympathy – or, as I've said, amusement; audience reaction varied there. But to have them both out of order was just possibly a touch vulgar, and altered the image somewhat. (A bad leg can, under fictionally romantic circumstances, conceivably have a bit of spurious glamour to it; but bad legs are altogether different!) Be that as it may, I was on the receiving end of many genuinely kind enquiries about my ear (just one), my head, my noises, my bells, my hum – were they trying to tell me something else? – and, most ominous of all, my Er . . . Um . . . Trouble. Never my ears!

But in the end, what does that matter? At the time one is struck chiefly by how kind people are to enquire at all; and that is the burden of my song here. However much those around you feel that they should tone down their responses because they may think you are over-playing your part, or even losing your marbles, it is wonderfully helpful if they can overcome their inner doubts about you, realise that although you look as healthy as you've ever done you are going through sheer hell, and offer themselves up, for five minutes even, as a listener – a buffer against the sound-storm.

One group of the world's tinnitus sufferers is unfortunately never able to enjoy the services of such a listener, or even of someone who will explain the dreadful mystery to them. Animals.

We used to have two cats, dear tabby moggies of no great price, but with charming and different personalities of their own. Katie lived to be seventeen, and was stone deaf towards the end. Boo-Boo died when she was eight, and I'm quite sure that she'd had to put up with some degree of deafness, and tinnitus, which were perhaps responsible for her sudden end.

She was admittedly a highly strung, nervous little thing, unlike her more stolid and supercilious companion, but nervousness alone wouldn't seem to account for a strange habit she developed for the last months of her life. At the time, I didn't guess what it might be, when I used to watch her with bewilderment, because it was another six months before I had tinnitus myself; but she would sometimes wake up from a sleep, look astonished, scared and baffled all together, and turn her head in a forlorn quest for something I couldn't see or hear. Meanwhile her ears would be twisting about in their feline direction-finding fashion. We could tell she was deaf in one ear, for though she had no trouble hearing in general, she couldn't hear in particular, having lost the ability to know where sounds came from. And she would dart in confusion to the person who wasn't calling her instead of the one who was. How much more muddling it must have been for her if she had tinnitus too. Eventually poor Boo-Boo made an error of this direction-finding kind on the road outside our house, and died of it.

I have in fact occasionally wondered if the virus I was told caused my woes had caused hers earlier. Six months would be a mightily long incubation period; but she was an affectionate cat to whom I gave many a cuddle. Or, seeing that Katie was deaf too, was it something to do with environment? No way of knowing now.

\* \* \*

7

There is nothing new under the sun, as we all know. And tinnitus must have been around ever since ears have. The School of Salerno pondered on the problem as long ago as the 13th century. And so did Alessandro Volta five hundred years or so later, when experimenting with the effect of an electric current on the ear, and discovering it sometimes suppressed tinnitus.

Famous people from Beethoven to Barbra Streisand have battled through their own sound barrages to reach the top of the tree. And perhaps similar barrages were responsible for a few revelations of the spiritual kind in years gone by. I know of an old lady who says her tinnitus takes the form of hymn tunes, and it may not be too a big a step from hearing religious music to receiving religious messages! But until recently people don't seem to have tried to pin down the causes of the complaint.

Getting to grips with causes is, even on the brink of the 21st century, easier said than done. So very many tinnitus cases totally defy diagnosis that it would be futile to picture each one as being neatly labelled and slotted into the right pigeon-hole. Thus the work of trying to treat the condition is baffling and complicated, especially as it is not actually an illness in itself. In fact, it's merely a symptom – of disease, damage, or disorder. And on all of this you'll find detailed information in 'Living with Tinnitus', which forms Part II of this book. You'll see then that, just as there is no all-embracing single cause of something as complex as tinnitus, there is no all-embracing 'blanket' cure. You can only cure a specific ailment; and tinnitus may arise from any one of literally dozens. You might be one of the lucky people in whom it is both identifiable and curable, but they aren't too thick on the ground. The rest of us have to think in terms of therapy.

The main instrument of tinnitus therapy has only been on the market in Britain since 1977, and that is the masker you wear like a hearing aid, a very versatile little piece of equipment with a frequency tailored to your own require-ments. (You get tested first!) Maskers are also dealt with thoroughly and scientifically in Part II, but they are worth a brief mention here. This is strictly a layman's account of the problems that can crop up along the route to acceptance, resignation, victory, or however you regard it. But the difficulties encountered when you ask a doctor about masking your tinnitus, or even when you are told that a masker would indeed help you, don't all come into a technical category.

The decision to mask or not to mask would normally be made by an E.N.T. consultant. You have to go through your own doctor first, of course, and occasionally you do find G.P.s who don't want to refer you to a consultant. Although it usually goes against the grain to do battle with the regular guardian of your family's health, you nevertheless have a perfect right to insist. But even specialists don't all come made to measure! You could just be unfortunate enough to be referred to one of the rare E.N.T. consultants who don't want to know about tinnitus; and it appears that there are a few of them still, strange as it may seem. Then your only recourse is to write to the BTA for information and assistance. But do please send along a stamped self-addressed envelope with your letter, for BTA exists on a very limited budget.

One other non-technical problem could arise if you are advised to have a masker: cost. At present there is no hard and fast ruling on whether or not you can get one through the National Health Service. Funding isn't on a centralised basis, but arranged by separate health authorities. So you have to find out how your own area stands where this is concerned. Prices you have to pay for maskers can vary, therefore, since different areas make different contributions. And some make none at all.

If you are recommended to a private supplier of maskers, the advice from all those who know is that you should never part with a large sum of money at the outset. You naturally have to pay your consultation fee – find out the amount first! – but you should be allowed to give the masker a short free trial before you agree to buy it; and only then hand over the money.

A final word on maskers: some people are put off them, or the idea of them, because they create another sound. One

more to add to the din within! Well, hope may be around the
corner. Experimental treatment is now going on at a Welsh
hospital for a new kind of masking, employing an inaudible
high frequency wavelength which masks out the tinnitus but
doesn't create noticeable noise of its own. A marvellous
thought for the future, if you can only hang on!

There are a lot of other valuable types of therapy,
meanwhile. Some are practical, scientifically based, others are
devices employed by the sufferers themselves – designs for
living, in effect. As far as practical methods of treatment go,
none so far seems to get rid of tinnitus completely, except in a
few rare cases. On a broader scale, they can sometimes give
relief from anxiety, and make the patient feel better in
general. If they eliminate stress they achieve a lot, for stress is
an interchangeable element with tinnitus; each can make the
other seem worse. Part II gives information about current
methods of therapeutic treatment, into which research is
being conducted in different centres nationwide. And, in
addition, counselling is now being considered as a possibility, in all the different forms it might take.

Telephone counselling, such as many organisations give,
like Samaritans, Alcoholics Anonymous and other help-lines,
is useful in that it provides instant comfort the very moment
you want it, when you're at the end of your tether. But
sometimes, for those who don't need to keep their problems
confidential, it can be more beneficial to talk them over with
other people like themselves, perhaps in a social atmosphere
similar to that of a BTA self-help group. (A list of local
self-help groups' addresses is on pages 131–37.) So group
counselling has also been considered. The third and maybe
the favourite idea is counselling in a private room inside a
hospital, with just one counsellor – who would be for
preference another tinnitus sufferer, surely the best kind of
listener. Counsellors wouldn't be *quite* the same as the
average 'other sufferer' like me! They wouldn't waste your
time regaling you with stories of their own troubles. They'd
be there to listen to yours.

On a more basic, do-it-yourself level, a lot of people find
keeping a bedside radio on all night very comforting when
they can't get off to sleep. This has its difficulties, of course, if

you share a bedroom. Likewise, though a loudly ticking clock might make tinnitus slightly better, a light sleeper on the other side of the bed could be kept awake all night long!

In the daytime, you'll be hardly likely to disturb anyone else by a bit of self-help; and the activities that people take up then, to get their minds away from their tinnitus, are as varied as human beings themselves. Yoga, aerobics, jogging – any type of exercise; you name it, someone is using it as tinnitus therapy.

A lot of us aren't really able to throw our bodies about, however, and quieter pursuits – which don't necessarily diminish noise but do diminish preoccupation with noise – are the order of the day then. One writer to the BTA said how much he had enjoyed a new-found hobby of bird-watching. He'd reorganised his garden so that the plants and shrubs attracted birds, and had built several bird-tables which now had countless regular customers. It had been a great source of pleasure to him. Other people have found other ways out, and the next chapter describes some of these.

Jack Ashley, who has to contend with severe deafness as well as tinnitus, says his recipe is to immerse himself in work, and then, when it's done, relax. And that's as good a therapy recipe as you'll get!

\* \* \*

## 8

It's always a help when you yourself are suffering, to discover what others in the same plight have to say about your mutual condition. I remember being ridiculously relieved to see one letter written to BTA's Postbag and published among their newsletters, asking why sleeping during the day made tinnitus so much worse. The Postbag answer confirmed this by saying that 80% of patients experienced the same thing. Suddenly I no longer felt a freak! Some of the letters written to BTA are intriguing as well as helpful to read, and here are a few extracts from them. They come under different classifications, which I've subdivided; and the first and perhaps most important of them is

*Comfort:*

'BTA is performing a useful service in making sufferers aware of one another, so that they do not feel so "peculiar," isolated and alone.'

'My doctor kindly lent me your Newsletter which he had obtained from another patient. Reading the letters does give a lot of comfort.'

'I have recently received a tinnitus masker and words cannot explain the difference it has made to me. I have more confidence in myself and can face each day in a better light.'

'May I say how much the BTA and my local Group have helped me? Without the existence of the BTA my life would be almost unbearable at times.'

Salvation of a sort has been worked out by one sector of the tinnitus community,

*The Philosophers:*

'I was at the Battle of the Somme which started on 1st July 1916. I was wounded on the 12th July at a place called Trones and taken to hospital. After I had been there two days this noise started in my left ear and has never left off since that date. It is like the old steam trains when they used to blow off steam . . . It is possible to live with it all this time as long as I don't think about it. I find it is worse when the weather is colder; in the summer it is not so bad.'

'I have become very anti-social because it is such a strain to make out what people are saying above the racket. So any social life crucifies me but, on my own, I can relax beautifully and to hell with everybody. Walking in the park – there's a lovely pond over the way and all the mallard, coots, greylags and moorhens *know* about tinnitus . . . I read, knit and haunt the art galleries. I garden though the earmould whistles when I bend . . . I can't enjoy radio or telly because of distortion but at least I sleep like a log and *never* take any dope.'

'I was becoming more and more wrapped up in the noises my ears were making. In desperation I answered an advert in the local paper for helpers for a disabled club and one evening with both hearing aids in I went to meet the members. This proved to be a turning point in my life, for since then I've become a pusher, [of wheelchairs!] made lots of friends and been on holiday with the club. So please take heart, tinnitus sufferers, it really does help yourself if you help others.'

'I find regular walks in the open air morning and evening quite useful. This does not cure tinnitus but certainly helps in reducing its severity and inducing easier sleep.'

'I avoid excessive stress and tension, eg heated arguments, quarrels, etc. I cultivate a calm, relaxed, philosophical attitude to life . . . I have trained myself to cultivate a driving, concentrated, powerful interest in an activity or subject close to my heart.'

One or two others have worked out their salvation on a simple and practical scale, such as one devotee of muesli and cold milk before bed, (highly successful it seems!) and another who sleeps in an elevated position with three pillows, and avers that you feel better if you smile.

The broadest view in the philosophical section was a plan for the future, one which nobody would dispute:

'In our cities of concrete, noise vibrates and reverberates in all directions. Sensitive people can *feel* the noise even when others are not aware that it's there . . . A man with a sledge hammer at one end of a concrete field will not only make his presence heard but felt too. But when the field is green-covered earth, then the noise is broken up and smothered. Let there be wide expanses of green in your concrete jungles, and you'll have a quieter, saner and more peaceful environment. This may help sufferers from tinnitus and prevent tinnitus arising in others.'

Another department is the one which proves you can't generalise. Your own particular poison might be
*One Man's Meat*:

On alcohol . . . 'I find whisky helps my tinnitus.'

'Alcohol makes my tinnitus worse.'

On radio . . . 'I have the radio on day and night as I love music and it's a great comfort to me.'

'The radio drives me to distraction and promotes noises rather than soothing them . . . I can almost feel the pain coming on.'

On acupuncture . . . 'I received eight treatments of acupuncture. During each session I experienced clicking noises in the offending ear, which pleased the acupuncturist. I cannot say that acupuncture cured my noises overnight, but

I think it reduced them slightly, and calmed me . . . I would recommend others to try acupuncture.'

'I have had £300 worth of treatment and it has not made any difference whatsoever.'

On hypnosis . . . 'At our [local group] meeting we were given a talk by the Hypnotherapist and one of our members was put under hypnosis. After the treatment she felt considerable relief and we have now learned she is able to reduce her tinnitus at will.'

'I was interested at the mention of hypnotherapy and that was the next thing I tried. I did not finish the course as after six expensive sessions my tinnitus was not even slightly improved.'

There are always some letters in categories of their own, such as the following:

'I have endured tinnitus for fifty years . . . and have donated my ears for research when I pass on. I have advised the necessary people – doctor, executor, relatives, etc. and carry a card stating all necessary details should death occur away from home.'

The Postbag answer (condensed) was: 'We wish it were possible to acquire more material like this. The problem is obtaining the ears soon enough. There are only a few specialist centres which can make use of this material but anyone interested should write to Professor Michaels, The Royal National Throat Nose and Ear Hospital, Gray's Inn Road, London, WC1.' (In case circumstances change, I should mention that this was written in March 1985).

The last word, or two, on the subject are those which we can only hope we won't be hearing much longer, in these more enlightened days:

'I took care not to complain to the doctors about this because the mere mention of "noises in the head" appeared to send them berserk. They were utterly frustrated by the condition.'

'My own G.P. does not seem to know tinnitus exists. Years ago a doctor told me it was my imagination.'

\* \* \*

It's not your imagination, though, is it? And hardly anyone nowadays believes it is. Tinnitus is a real sound, measurable in a few cases from outside, by special listening apparatus. And it's very important to keep in your mind the fact that no one can any longer write you off as a crank with a vivid imagination, just because you have a complaint which you alone can detect. There are other people, worldwide, with problems like yours and despair like you may feel at times. And, however much of a loner you are by nature, this must in the end be a comfort.

Statistically, it is surprising how few of its victims seek medical advice for tinnitus. It's estimated that roughly one person in ten who has it goes to the doctor about it; the other nine just put up with it. Which I suppose means that most of those who don't take it further are the lucky ones whose noises are mild enough to be only a vague nuisance. But that still leaves a lot of others, those who are undergoing the real thing – the sounds that can terrify by their intensity, particularly when they are new.

Even the most experienced doctors tend to regard the really persistent complainants (presumably from the second, less lucky group) as people prone to anxiety and depressive problems, maybe possessing types of personality that wouldn't be able to cope with even a low level of tinnitus.

This may indeed be true in some cases, but it does seem a very sweeping judgment. It can surely be a question of which came first, the chicken or the egg. It's easy to be cheerful and dismissive about it all, as I myself have found, when the noise isn't too obtrusive, yet impossible not to be anxious and depressed when the noise is shrieking at top volume. Who wouldn't be?

If you are among this sector, with a lot of troublesome sound to contend with, and you live alone or with no one sympathetic to talk to, it's worth trying to get out and mix with other people if you possibly can – in whatever way is open to you. You may have a full-time job, in which case you could see enough other people during the day to want a contrast in your spare time; but for many tinnitus sufferers the onset comes at approximately retirement age, just as things are quietening down outside.

So long as you're blessed with normal mobility, you can still find some part of that great outside which needs you, and in which you can receive solace in return – as the deaf lady writing in the previous chapter, who takes out disabled people in wheelchairs, discovered. I think if I'd lived alone, I'd have tried first to go to a BTA group, if there had been one nearby. Otherwise, I'd have looked about like she did for some voluntary work to do which entailed being with others with different needs from my own. However tiring, difficult or even saddening the task might have proved to be, it would still have been a useful kind of therapy – in an instance such as hers, useful to more than just me.

Though your results may not come to anything, there's nothing to stop you from trying to help yourself to slightly quieter ears around the home. I found it beneficial at one stage to make notes of everything I did during the day, and mark my tinnitus level against each detail. At another period I just marked the day's level; I found it recently when looking through my 1981 diary for something else, and couldn't at first think what all the strange abbreviations signified! The system had its uses, for I would analyse it all at the end of a fortnight to see if any pattern emerged, of things to do and things to avoid. On rare occasions I did see some pattern, and acted on its indications.

At any rate, if one thing doesn't work for you, try something else, the complete opposite, perhaps. Keep experimenting. To some extent – without trying really weird 'cures' or diets, of course – be your own guide and mentor. You are there, on the spot, knowing exact reactions the moment they occur.

Studying reactions, you can, alas, end up every bit as confused as you started out. One man wrote to BTA that when he was under pressure, of work or play – and, as he commented, the adrenalin was flowing – the noises went away, to return worse than ever once he relaxed. (Just like me, so I found that part very interesting!) Yet ironically, once he began to lead a quieter life in general, the noise quietened down in general too. Bored with inactivity, he later took on more responsibilities again, only to find his tinnitus pattern back at Square One. So, as he said, his experiences were rather conflicting!

Wherever you get to in this respect, it's an accepted fact that, as in so many other types of distress, time really does make everything seem better. Which may mean that eventually it isn't just a case of your mind and body having to make all the adjustments on their own. The tinnitus may do a bit of adjusting itself.

The seven years or so since its onset has seen a change in my own tinnitus, not just accounted for by altered perception – for on the odd occasions when it decides to go full blast again it offends me as much as it ever did. But familiarity breeds contempt, and it doesn't frighten me any more.

Aspects of having tinnitus still present a lasting annoyance, however. The absence of birdsong in my life, mainly – for the virus that set my over-active hair-cells vibrating in their beastly inner ear dance also destroyed my upper range of sound. Though even then perhaps it's not all bad. I am spared the dawn chorus.

On the whole my noises now range from a shrill ensemble of police whistles to the gentle leg-rubbing of a family of little cicadas on a Mediterranean summer night. And it can at times even disappear completely, for as much as an hour or so. Once in a while I still get the oddest oscillations, like the visual ones I had earlier, four to a heartbeat – but bodily this time, from top to toe. A strange feeling, rather as if I've been turned into a sort of muted road drill, and more than a little disturbing when I'm lying in bed at night! It's a lot less dizzy-making than the visual variety, but not exactly comfortable, even so.

Nevertheless it's all very much better than it was, and most of the time I can dismiss it from my mind. I stop and listen sometimes, realise it's still there, then shrug it off again. To illustrate, two years ago we moved house; I was put onto the National Health Service list of a doctor who didn't have my card to refer to, and was asked if I had any ongoing problems. Completely forgetting the existence of my tinnitus, I breezily said no. That's how much it bothers me now.

I know it could go bad on me again some time. Instability of any sort is unreliable. And as it once got better, I'm not blind to the fact that it could just as easily get worse. If it does, I'll always remember that I got through it the last time, and try to meet it with courage. In any case, I shall never lose hope.

And that's the point, in the end. The message you are given ought to be one of hope, I feel. Perhaps for some rare people it may be preferable not to long for miracles, but to reach instead a state of acceptance as soon as possible, on the assumption that their troubles will always be with them in the same way, never diminishing one iota. But for others – most of us, surely? – it must help to have a little germ of hope seeing us through from one day to the next.

Research is going on all the time, and who can really tell in advance when the big discoveries are going to come? They may take longer than the ten years and beyond, which are at present forecast. But they may not. After all, the dream of space travel caught up with reality faster than anyone would have ever believed possible back in the first half of this century. And the dream of going to bed at night and laying one's head upon a silent pillow again may not be so wildly unrealistic, either.

And on your own individual plane there is always hope, too. Never mind if doctors tell you that you'll never get the slightest bit better. They are knowledgeable, yes. But they're not omniscient. And tinnitus isn't so thoroughly known or understood (as they'll readily admit) as most other ear conditions.

I can only assure you that my own nasty sounds have abated considerably over the years that I've been lumbered with them – though I was told that they wouldn't. I am not yet deaf enough for it to be a social disadvantage – though I was told that I would be. I did not turn out to have Ménière's Disease – though I was told that I had. One way and another, the body sometimes accidentally triumphs over the dogmas that the experts have laid down for it. If that minor miracle can happen to me, it can happen to you.

But even if it doesn't and nothing is eased, ever, for so much as a split second, there has got to come a time when you stand still, take stock, and think of what appalling and shattering disabilities some brave people manage to conquer – with marvellous fortitude and the ultimate tranquillity that a sense of achievement brings. And you realise that, horrible though it is, even severe and permanent tinnitus isn't by any means the direst weapon that Fate can use to strike you down.

# PART II

# Living with Tinnitus

by

LESLIE SHEPPARD

*This book is dedicated
to all those for whom
Silence is a Stranger*

*Leslie Sheppard*

# Author's Notes

Like so many others, with the onset of tinnitus a few years ago I submitted to all the orthodox tests only to be blandly told 'nothing can be done'.

My first reaction was one of anger and frustration and I began to search libraries and book lists for any literature on the subject that I might more fully understand just what had hit me. But I found that no book on the subject existed.

After a while I discovered the British Tinnitus Association. Merely to find that I was not alone with my problem enabled me to come to terms with it more readily. I found the B.T.A. newsletters of especial interest, and gradually I was able to obtain various internationally produced medical papers and reports of trials on tinnitus.

As a writer I then began to publish some magazine articles on tinnitus in an effort to draw more public attention to the condition and to the work of the B.T.A. This required quite an amount of research and the more I probed, the more absorbing the subject became, and it was not so long before the idea of producing a book, which would hopefully be of use to other sufferers, became uppermost in my mind.

The result lies before you. Alas, it offers no magical cure for tinnitus, for so far no cure exists. But it is my sincere wish that it may give a sufferer some knowledge of the various aspects of the condition and the difficulties of research, together with some suggestions for self-help, and thus by giving more understanding of the condition may assist him or her to come to terms with it more readily.

My sincere thanks go to Pamela Kennedy, Co-ordinator of the British Tinnitus Association, and latterly to David Wiggins her successor, for the willing help they have both so kindly extended to me in the preparation of this book; particularly for permission to quote so freely from the many helpful and interesting letters with expert replies that have appeared in the B.T.A. Newsletters. In these, I feel that readers are given the opportunity to feel they are actually 'sitting in' on the consultations of other sufferers, with so many of whom they will easily be able to identify.

On the Psychological Aspects of Tinnitus as with Treatment by Hypnosis, I found available bibliography sadly lacking, and wish to express my most grateful thanks to both Richard Hallam and Hellmut Karle who so readily came to my aid with their excellent contributions on these two important aspects.

Whilst the root causes of tinnitus and much more have yet to be fully understood, no-one should be content with negative advice; there are devices and means available that can help so many sufferers, and sources to which one can turn for advice and practical help in so many different ways.

Additionally, there is much that can be achieved by self-help in an endeavour to at least alleviate to a certain extent this distressing condition – until that happy day dawns when a breakthrough is made by those now engaged in so earnestly searching for a cure.

LESLIE SHEPPARD

# The Current Background

Mr Jonathan Hazell F.R.C.S., the Consultant Neuro-otologist in charge of the Tinnitus Clinic at the Royal Ear Hospital, University College, is the R.N.I.D.'s Medical Adviser.

He has pioneered tinnitus research in this country, having been appointed by the R.N.I.D. about twelve years ago to undertake research into Deafness and Tinnitus. As a result of his co-operation with Mr George Williams, an elelectrical engineer, together with Professor Jack Vernon of the Kreage Hearing Laboratory, Portland, Oregon, the first prototype tinnitus masker was introduced in this country in 1977. Tinnitus maskers have since become available on the National Health Service on the recommendation of E.N.T. consultants. Currently the D.H.S.S. is evaluating a report which it has commissioned on the place of maskers in the treatment of tinnitus. The project was undertaken by three centres – The Royal Ear Hospital in London, the Institute of Hearing Research in Nottingham, and the Royal National Throat Nose & Ear Hospital in London, the consultants concerned being Mr Jonathan Hazell, Dr Ross Coles, and Dr Dai Stephens.

Mr Hazell is also engaged in the Cochlear Implant programme at the Royal Ear Hospital. Patients selected for this advanced form of micro-surgery, which aims to provide sounds which will act as an aid to lip reading for post-lingually profoundly deaf people, will in future be patients who additionally suffer from tinnitus. The hope is that ultimately this form of surgery may be used to help other tinnitus sufferers, although it must be emphasised that this still lies in the future.

# I

# Introductory

Most unwanted sounds can engender considerable annoyance and stress, especially when experienced over a period, but at least there is an end to such noises at some time. Yet for some people there is no such end. Day and night, noise is with them. There is no escape.

Such is the unremitting misery of those who suffer from the ear condition known as tinnitus, and it has been authoritatively estimated that in Great Britain alone 20%–25% of the population suffer from bothersome tinnitus: ranging from an occasional nuisance, to a small percentage who would be inclined to suicidal tendencies because of this affliction.

Tinnitus affects sufferers to varying degrees, and the noises they hear likewise vary considerably. Unfortunately, so far no positive cure has been found for this distressing condition, and indeed the all-too-usual medical advice that the majority of sufferers can expect to receive is that they must just learn to live with it.

It is a most depressing and essentially private misery. It is every bit as difficult to bear as some of the more visible ills to which human flesh is heir, yet one can meet a dozen fellow-sufferers in the course of a single day without even being aware of their hidden hell.

## THE HISTORY OF TINNITUS

Tinnitus is no present-day malady triggered off by the noise and pace of modern living, as some people imagine. There is also evidence that the symptom has been prevalent since earliest times in both Egypt and Mesopotamia. Throughout history there has always been a division of opinion as to whether it is an illness in its own right or a symptom of some other condition. We know today that it is certainly not a complaint in itself but a symptom of a wide variety and usually microscopic abnormalities affecting the mechanism of hearing.

In early times, when doctors were also priests, they clung to the ancient belief that all illness was caused by an evil spirit which needed to be driven from the body in order to effect relief, whereon hapless patients were required to swallow remedies so obnoxious that the evil spirits would vacate their bodies in haste.

Pliny the Elder referred to tinnitus in his compendium of remedies for ear complaints both 'traditional' and 'orthodox' in which he gave treatments for tinnitus. Such treatments included the taking of foam from the mouth of a horse, mother's milk, and donkey dung. Such bizarre remedies were in use almost to the start of the nineteenth century.

Treatment for man's many ills has taken odd turnings during the long history of medicine. There exists an account of an eminent physician of his time, Dr Hans Sloane, administering viper broth to a patient in 1690, and of the Royal Society being requested to report on the medicinal value of unicorn horn! Whilst on the list of remedies for various complaints existing even a century later there appear such items as oil from ants and wolves, animal excreta, fox lungs, spider webs, swallow nests, wood lice, and even the skulls of executed criminals.

Near the close of the seventeenth century Du Verney wrote one of the first important books on ear disease, and gave considerable coverage to the subject of tinnitus, which even then may well have been at as high an incidence as it is today. Many were the cures, both herbal and otherwise, for earache, loss of hearing and tinnitus, and these may well have appeared to have been effective by sole reason of the fact that they reassured the patient that at least *something* was being done to deal with the cause of the problem and thus probably made it easier to accept the symptom.

Much of the treatment for tinnitus meted out in the past certainly seems to have been more psychological than medical in its application. The Babylonians sang incantations, begging the 'ghost' causing the tinnitus to leave the patient's ear. Sometimes certain spells would be accompanied by the application of oils or the administration of purgatives – the latter was always a great favourite for most ills.

The Indian Annamites believed that actual hearing depended on a tiny animal inside the ear, and if this became involved in a fight with another similar animal the result was tinnitus. Their favourite remedy was to fumigate the offending ear with smoke from a burning snake skin.

The Greeks, who believed in the humoral theory of Anaxagoras (circa BC 500), were quite certain that tinnitus was caused by an upset in the 'humours' and gave the usual purgatives, applying oils to the outer part of the ear.

Later the earliest surgery for tinnitus took up the theory from the Greeks which suggested that tinnitus was the outcome of air being trapped within the ear. It was thought that surgery which allowed this trapped air to escape would cure the tinnitus, which of course it did not.

The application of electricity was instituted by Wibel and others in the mid-eighteenth century, but alas again such efforts met with failure.

In more recent times attitudes changed within the medical profession with the frank admittance that for many sufferers from tinnitus there was no known cure. The best that could be done was to discover ways of relieving the effects of the condition on the patient. By and large, this attitude has remained. There is still no general cure and unfortunately in Great Britain the problem of tinnitus has been accorded a very low level of priority – a fact conceded by the Institute of Hearing Research.

## THE INCIDENCE OF TINNITUS

According to the National Centre for Health Statistics in America some 32% of the whole population of the U.S.A. have suffered from tinnitus at some time or other in their lives, with around 6% of these people suffering a degree of the condition so severe as to be debilitating.

So far as Great Britain is concerned, it has been

authentically estimated that some 300,000 of the population suffer from tinnitus to the extent that it destroys normal life for them.

In the examination of 2,000 of his patients taken consecutively, one specialist has stated that 1700 of these patients suffered from tinnitus to one degree or another, and the condition is most prevalent between the ages of 51 and 60, increasing up to around the age of 70, after which it appears to decline. For some unknown reason it has been found to be far more common in women than in men.

## TYPES OF TINNITUS

Objective tinnitus is in the normal way the type with little connection with hearing and is associated with roughness in the joint of the jaw situated immediately in front of the ear, or with contractions in the muscles of the soft palate and irregularities in the blood flow of the larger arteries leading to the head.

Subjective tinnitus refers to a condition which manifests itself in a sensation of sound without any relevant external stimulus, and is far and away the more common. It is often, though not always, associated with a hearing loss and somewhat ironically this constant sensation of sound can affect even those with no hearing whatever. The condition when existing to a serious degree can be a very grave problem to the sufferer, yet to others there is no audible nor visible sign that anything is wrong.

We shall be looking further on at the attempts that have been made in the treatment of tinnitus, but it must be emphasised that in the great majority of cases any such treatments can at present only be palliative, since no general cure is known. Alas these attempts are little more than bandages for they do not heal the wound.

All this goes to highlight the very real and urgent need for far more funding to be made available for tinnitus research and a higher level of priority afforded it by those in high places.

## TINNITUS & PSYCHOLOGY

There is little doubt that any tinnitus sufferer can easily fall
victim to considerable psychological problems, finding but
little response, interest, or care from the professionals to
whom he or she usually turns.

As with so many other conditions, the mere fact of
receiving 'treatment' is a psychological help, but all too often
sufferers from tinnitus stand alone in this respect, receiving
no treatment and no hope, their plight apparently ignored. In
such conditions frustration alone can set up a strong
psychological response. It is a known fact that tinnitus can
actually affect the personality of the sufferer considerably,
and it has further been proved that through the mutual action
between psychological and physiological elements in times of
stress the intensity of the tinnitus becomes all the greater.

## TINNITUS & SURGERY

The onset of tinnitus *can* signal the existence of a tumour
within the auditory system, and such a case does of course
require surgery and in carrying out such surgery the surgeon
might well cure the tinnitus. However, such a case cannot
really be looked upon as surgery for alleviation of tinnitus.

In the past certain surgical attempts have been made with
the object of relieving tinnitus, but the success rates do not
provide a very good track record.

The existing general medical opinion seems to be against
surgical interference until much more is known regarding the
condition, and especially since any such operation carried out
with existing knowledge could well adversely affect more
successful and enlightened treatment in the future.

## RESEARCH DIFFICULTIES

There is little doubt that subjective tinnitus is a symptom of a
variety of different and often microscopic abnormalities, and
this may well be the reason why the sounds that people hear

vary so much. It is virtually impossible to treat a symptom
without *complete* knowledge of the underlying cause, and this
is one of the main reasons why medical research has yet to
find the true path that will lead to a cure. Yet if and when that
cure comes, it will most certainly not be in the form of 'a little
pill to make it all better' – the condition is so obviously too
complex for that.

Even the level of sound heard by each individual sufferer
varies according to their own description of it, for it is difficult
for anyone to equate the level of a sound within the head to
that of a sound in the outside world. However, Professor
Feldman of Heidelberg has used masking bands of 'white
noise' at differing intensities in an attempt to measure the
actual level of loudness experienced by a sufferer, with
considerable success in this connection.

Emissions of sound have lately been shown to occur in
many people with tonal tinnitus, but these may only be heard
with an intrameatal microphone and powerful amplifier. It is
thought that these emissions arise from sound from within
the cochlea. Such sounds are quite different from, and should
not be confused with, those noises produced by muscular
clicks and so on within the jaw, which are often possible to
hear through even a stethoscope.

## II

# The Sounds of Tinnitus

The word 'tinnitus' literally means a 'ringing sound' and in many cases it is precisely this, but the noises reported by sufferers differ considerably. Here are just a few:

> The sound of running water
> The sound of the sea, as though a shell is held to the ear
> The hiss of escaping steam
> A high pitched screaming noise
> The sound of a swarm of bees
> A sound like a cistern refilling
> Like ping-pong balls playing around in the head
> Rather like the sound of an air-raid warning
> Like a diesel lorry ticking over in the next street
> A clicking sound
> A buzzing sound
> A low throbbing hum
> Like a bird chirping
> A fizzing sound
> A constant whistling noise
> A sound like a heart beat (pulsatile tinnitus)

Doubtless many readers will be able to identify their tinnitus with one of the above sounds, others to add to the list. Nearly everything that is known concerning the sounds of tinnitus must of necessity come from the reports of patients, and naturally one patient's description of the same sound often does not match that of another. Obviously a standard set of questions should be asked before any true research on this could be undertaken.

Likewise on the question of 'where does the noise appear to come from?' many reports are confusing. Is it in one ear? Is it in both? Is it from inside the head? Unfortunately neither the quality nor the actual sound of tinnitus is any guide at all to its origin.

Researchers are faced with a wide range of descriptions of the sounds of tinnitus from various sufferers. How much more valuable it would be to have a completely non-verbal method of assessment of the actual sounds heard. In this way perhaps it might be easier to establish a connection between the tinnitus quality and site of origin if such a connection exists.

There also appears to be great need for further research into the characteristics of tinnitus. For example, it might be in one ear only; it might be in both ears each giving similar sounds; it could be in both ears with characteristics similar but not of equal loudness. It could be at one frequency in one ear and at another frequency in the other. Lack of information on such important points as this may well be the reason for the failure of such devices as tinnitus maskers and tinnitus instruments with some sufferers.

## B.T.A. TAPE RECORDING

An excellent tape recording which includes the simulated sounds of tinnitus is available from the British Tinnitus Association price £1.50.

*Letter:* Just knowing that there are so many other sufferers from tinnitus has literally saved my reason. Like so many others I thought I was either going mad fast or else had cancer of the brain. I am so relieved to know that I am only one of millions who have thought similarly. My dear husband has never been able to imagine what it is like to have a whistle blowing in one's ear incessantly, 24 hours a day, and he is quite shattered and much more sympathetic since he heard the B.T.A. Tape.

*Letter:* I have suffered from tinnitus for the last five years . . . coming on after a very bad throat and catarrh. I have a high pitched hum like a TV set left on after the programmes have finished. This I have learned to live with, but it is much worse after a cold.
*Reply:* The sort of tinnitus from which you suffer is extremely common and probably not associated with any catarrh or middle ear condition. However, having a blockage in the middle ear after a cold makes any kind of tinnitus worse.

*Letter:* I have deafness and tinnitus which has been quite controllable until now. I have a hearing aid which really does not 'aid' but gives a contact with the hearing world, any noise being more acceptable than the internal racket. Recently my tinnitus has become intolerable – a high pitched scream and a throbbing first in one ear and then in the other, plus a lower slightly musical hum. I have recently had a virus infection and was also pulled over by my dog which gave me a shock. Could either of these be the reason for my increased tinnitus?

*Reply:* It is not likely that there is any connection between your accident and your other problem. However the virus infection may have temporarily affected the tinnitus level which does go up and down with stress and strain.

*Letter:* My form of tinnitus is a constant repetition of musical notes . . . what has worried me for some time is that as soon as I lie down the noises become worse and I develop terrific headaches. It seems that the fluid from the spine flows into the brain when in a recumbent position. On rising and when I am in an upright position, it slowly disperses . . . does the spinal fluid have any effect on tinnitus or deafness generally?

*Reply:* Tinnitus often becomes worse when a sufferer lies down. This is partly because you lie down in a quiet environment where the tinnitus is not masked by environmental sounds. The terrific headaches are usually due to muscle tension over the neck and scalp muscles. It is possible there is a change in pressure in the inner ear which affects tinnitus since you are right in thinking that the cerebrospinal fluid in the brain can sometimes connect with the perilymph fluid in the inner ear. I am afraid there is no solution for this problem apart from sleeping in a more upright position. Have you tried using two or three pillows?

*Letter:* A writer complained of repetitive noises in the ear and you replied that if she can hear words or sentences, then this is usually another condition. It might help further understanding if I wrote and told you that patient may indeed be suffering from yet another type of background noise, maybe fairly unusual, and so not added to the list. I have a noise, amongst all the others that are there every minute of the day and night, in my right ear. It certainly sounds like voices, because the noise rises and falls like speech, rather like having a telephone receiver to the ear but unable to catch what the person is saying. Although I have tinnitus in both ears, I only get this type in the right ear along with hissing and buzzing. One cannot help but think that with this particular type of noise a sufferer could easily think he or she was going 'dotty'.

*Reply:* I think your comments will be extremely helpful to other tinnitus sufferers. I think the noise you describe is tinnitus but it is being produced fairly high up in the auditory tract. It is very difficult to say where the borderline between an abnormality in the hearing system and a change in the brain (which could possibly be called a borderline psychiatric condition) meets. One has to look at each case in detail and decide. But from the information you give it is unlikely you are 'going dotty'.

*Letter:* Until the end of last year I was employed as a teacher but because of very severe deafness have taken early retirement . . . like many severely deaf people I suffer from tinnitus, one symptom of which is a continual and high pitched sound in the left ear. But what is even more alarming and disconcerting is the popping that occurs in the vicinity of the right ear. The effect is difficult to describe. Not only do I hear the pop, I can actually feel it, and at times it can be a most terrifying and violent sensation. It appears to me that the ear is back-firing. Is this due to over-exertion? But that cannot be so because it can occur during sleep, and although I may not awaken, I am aware that it is taking place. However, I understand that this could be another manifestation of tinnitus. If so, it can be accepted. If not, then there must be another explanation.

*Reply:* It sounds as if you have two rather separate but equally common conditions. The high-pitched continual sound is what is commonly described as tinnitus. The other popping sensations are caused by the eustachian tube opening and closing, sometimes when you swallow. Certainly exercise can make this worse and if the ear drum becomes a bit limp, as it sometimes does as the years go by, it can amplify the sounds of popping. It has absolutely no significance apart from being tiresome and annoying. An ear specialist would be able to confirm my suggestion after proper examination.

*Letter:* Although I have had tinnitus in my right ear for many years it does not affect me too seriously, as outside noises blot it out. But during the last three years I have experienced on occasion a single tone ring go right through my ear lasting a second or two. It can happen in either ear . . . what has caused it, and what is it?

*Reply:* Everybody has this short-duration high-pitched tinnitus from time to time and I think it has become just a little bit more common in your case. We are not quite sure what causes it, but it does seem to be due to over activity of the hair cells in the inner ear. There is no underlying medical problem that needs to be treated. I know that many people feel that these noises are caused by some psychiatric illness or a tumour in the head. This is simply not the case.

## SPONTANEOUS OTOACOUSTIC EMISSIONS (O.A.E's)

A number of investigators have experimented by the insertion of a very sensitive microphone into the ears of patients, and been most surprised to discover that it is far from uncommon for quite normal ears to emit what are known as spontaneous otoacoustic emissions (or O.A.E.s) normally far too weak in signal strength to be picked up by ordinary means, even with a stethoscope. Curiously, again, most of these O.A.E.s cannot be heard by the people possessing them, and can thus in no way be referred to as tinnitus – a *conscious* knowledge of sound in the head.

This then gives us (a) the usual type of objective tinnitus arising from some structure in the middle or inner ear, head, jaw or neck, (b) the normally discussed subjective tinnitus which is the sensation of sounds without any external stimulus, and (c) those sounds which are thought to be emitted by the cochlea which can be heard in the hearing canal by sensitive microphones but are not audible to the person who has them – viz. O.A.E.s.

There *have* been cases reported of tinnitus sufferers who can actually hear the tonal sound of the O.A.E.s heard by those using a sensitive microphone in their ear. Yet quite a few have had a number of unheard O.A.E.s occasionally accompanied by just one of which they were conscious.

In one experiment twenty normal-hearing subjects were examined, resulting in five with O.A.E.s audible to the testers yet none of these sounds audible to their owners, and strangely in another test on some three dozen people over twenty O.A.E.s were discovered, none of which corresponded to any reported tinnitus; with a further sixteen people examined who complained of tinnitus of varying kinds no O.A.E.s at all were discovered!

In an experiment conducted in 1981 on people who had answered a newspaper invitation asking for tinnitus sufferers, four out of ten of these people were found to have an O.A.E. corresponding to the tinnitus of which they complained. However, it must be added that the tinnitus found in these volunteers was not of a particularly severe type. The four subjects in whom the O.A.E. was found to be identical to

the sound that they were actually hearing is a strong
indication that the two matters are closely related – yet not in
every way.

In pitch matching tests the pitch of the tinnitus and the
O.A.E. have both been obliterated by the adjustment of the
level of an external sound, and if alterations are made in the
air pressure in the outer-ear canal it is found that the pitch of
the tinnitus and the O.A.E. both rise correspondingly.

Although considerable tonal content is found in actual
tinnitus sounds, it is of interest to mention that O.A.E.s have
not been heard in this category, being rougher and noisier
and rather indicating that in effect O.A.E.s are actually noise
bands.

## PULSATILE TINNITUS

Pulsatile tinnitus is the type of tinnitus resulting in a
pulsating noise nearly always in precise rhythm with the
sufferer's heartbeat, and accounts for some 20% of cases. It
can be caused by the ear being aware of the flow of blood
through the larger vessels going into the head, or can be blood
pulsing noisily through the tiny vessels of the inner ear.
Fortunately this type of tinnitus does not indicate any serious
condition, and masking is the most helpful treatment.

> *Letter:*   I have the same trouble as the writer in newsletter 15 i.e.
> 'swish, swish,' in time with my pulse. In your reply you said the
> cause of the noise was a slight roughening in one of the big blood
> vessels in the head. Perhaps you could tell me whether this
> condition is likely to worsen or whether it remains the same for
> the rest of one's life.
> *Reply:*   Usually this kind of pulsatile tinnitus stays much the
> same, although many people find they adapt to it, and it becomes
> less of a problem to them as time goes on. Masking can often help.

## RECRUITMENT

We are all familiar with the old joke in which an actor shouts into the earpiece of a 'deaf' person with the result that they jump dramatically, to the delight of the audience. Alas, deafness is an eternal joke to all those who do not suffer from it.

A phenomenon of both deafness and tinnitus is that very often people suffer from an abnormally rapid rate of growth of loudness. Loud sounds are heard well above threshold. Although the ear may not hear quiet sounds it is unable to tolerate really loud ones. This phenomenon is known as recruitment and occurs in up to 15% of tinnitus sufferers.

There are at present two ways of coping with the difficulty. Firstly, a hearing aid that is fitted with a form of compression or automatic gain control, similar to that used on tape recorders to avoid too high a volume in recording. Such can usually only be obtained privately. Unfortunately a certain amount of distortion can be produced in quiet sounds, although in the latest instruments attention has been focussed on this. Secondly, in the case of those suffering from Ménière's Disease many may find considerable relief from this annoying condition by wearing ear plugs, either of the soft type which expand, or a custom-built mould similar to that of some hearing aids which occlude the ear (used without the sound channel of course). Enquiry should be made from firms specialising in hearing aids, or the audiology department of your local hospital. But it must be stressed that neither method is absolutely perfect.

*Letter:* Last August I suddenly developed tinnitus and severe deafness in one ear. When some weeks later I was told that I had a blood vessel jammed in the eardrum and that there was no cure, I didn't know how I was going to live with the situation. A second opinion produced the same diagnosis although both consultants admitted it was speculation.

The second consultant suggested I contact the British Tinnitus Association and this gave an immediate boost to my morale and enabled me to get in touch with a manufacturer of tinnitus maskers. The masker was not of use to me because for quite some time noise had been painful and although this has settled down to mere discomfort, it is outside noise which seems to aggravate the tinnitus.

The manufacturer put me in touch with a hearing aid centre who had a hearing aid made up for me to conform to my audiogram, although the part of my hearing which should hear words has, I was told, been destroyed. This aid prevents any noise above a certain number of decibels from entering my ear.

I understand it is unusual for tinnitus sufferers to be sensitive to noise, but I thought that if any readers have the same condition they might like to know that considerable relief can be obtained from this kind of hearing aid.

*Reply:* Many tinnitus sufferers experience recruitment or sensitivity to loud noise, so what your consultant told you was not strictly true. It underlines the problem that we meet with all the time, that so few people know anything about this condition having chosen to ignore it for so long. It has been known since 1935 that a hearing aid can give considerable relief to tinnitus and is something that everyone with hearing loss and tinnitus should try. If you have a hearing loss and suffer from sensitivity to loud noise, it is possible to be helped by a hearing aid. The aid however has to be adjusted so that the maximum amount of sound that it feeds into the ear – for instance when loud sounds are picked up by the microphone – does not cause pain by exceeding your level of discomfort. The way in which this adjustment is carried out will depend on the type of aid that you have.

*Letter:* Would you consider it advisable for a person with loud tinnitus and added recruitment to restrict their exposure to what to them seems to be too loud and too long a duration of chatter and noise which results in a head of noise and tension bordering on pain? I feel I must be allowed to say 'no' to invitations and meetings which would be a trial.

*Reply:* About 10% to 15% of people with tinnitus suffer from recruitment or loudness discomfort. Sometimes this means that when they are exposed to loud noise their tinnitus gets worse. Many people find the tinnitus gets worse if they are in a noisy environment, because this is often a stressful environment. It is always very difficult to work out whether the discomfort is due to the increased tinnitus level or the noise. As a general rule no one should expose themselves to noise that is painful and if this is a relatively low level because of recruitment, then that is the level that they should avoid exposing themselves to. I often recommend the wearing of ear plugs . . . and learning to say 'no' is something we all have to do. Many of us are not very good at it. Clearly, if we have something that makes our life more difficult, like tinnitus or recruitment or both, then we should say 'no' more often than we might otherwise.

# III

# The Causes of Tinnitus

Causes behind the onset of tinnitus are both numerous and diverse. There may on the one hand be obstruction (i.e. wax in the outer or middle ears) or thickening of the bone around the window transmitting sound from the middle to the inner ear (otosclerosus). Or the condition may be brought on by the pathological changes caused by extreme noise or by the use of certain drugs. Again there may be actual physical distortion of the hearing mechanism such as usually causes the tinnitus accompanying Ménière's Disease.

In searching for the possible causes of tinnitus one comes across many theories, some possible, some questionable. Some ideas are merely common intuition and are accepted as true by far too many because of the lack of any more expert information being available.

## MULTIPLE ORIGINS

No one stated cause for the onset of tinnitus can be all embracing, for so obviously the origins of the condition are multiple. Just occasionally the origin of a person's tinnitus has been discovered – this is especially possible in the case of the type that can be heard by others (i.e. objective tinnitus) but the actual cause in the great majority of cases still remains something of a mystery.

## IMPORTANCE OF THE SITE OF ORIGIN

There is thus much research still to be undertaken in this particular field, for if the site of origin in each tinnitus sufferer could be established beyond all doubt, then the correct type of treatment for that specific cause would be more likely to be found. It is precisely the present ignorance concerning the site of origin that is so obviously the root cause of the present unsatisfactory position regarding correct treatment. Letters from sufferers contain a variety of suggestions as to the likely cause of their own particular tinnitus.

## ACCIDENTS

There are frequent reports of tinnitus starting following an accident involving head injury, and this type of tinnitus is usually of a high pitched quality. Nearly all such cases find masking the most efficient treatment available at present.

## AUDIBLE BURGLAR ALARMS

*Letter:* I have worked for the past three and a half years for a Burglar Alarm Company in close proximity to a demonstration model of a burglar alarm system, left switched on day and night. This equipment, an Ultratec Ultrasonic Detector emits very high frequencies that are audible up close. I have recently discovered that the manufacturers recommend that this equipment be switched off when personnel are on the premises as it may have an irritating effect on hearing.

It would appear from this that the manufacturers have some information concerning the effect of their equipment which has not been made generally available; otherwise they would not have issued such a warning. The offending equipment has now been removed and replaced by a model which emits a higher frequency (not audible when close) presumably to overcome this defect. Is it logical that any equipment emitting certain high frequencies (as television, stereo radio) could trigger off tinnitus? I began to suffer from tinnitus in 1977 when I was 26 and still have it.

*Reply:* Frankly, I do not know the answer. But it is conceiveable that there may be something in this.

## CATARRH

*Letter:* Since a prolonged attack of severe catarrh, during which both eustachian tubes became blocked, I have suffered from tinnitus. Neither the E.N.T. specialist nor my doctor will give an opinion on whether the tinnitus is caused by catarrh. Can you tell me if this could be the cause?

*Reply:* Just occasionally, tinnitus is caused by catarrh. The eustachian tube fails to open properly and there is a problem with the middle ear. However, this is far less common than inner ear tinnitus which does not respond to catarrh treatment.

Catarrh actually means fluid running from the nose, as experienced with a heavy cold. A feeling of blockage in the nose which people describe as catarrh does not usually affect middle ear function. Objective tests are now available for eustachian function and middle ear pressure and if these are normal the cause of your tinnitus is unlikely to be due to anything in the nose.

## DISCOS

The risk of hearing loss from the constant loud noise of the modern discos has also been a source of some research, and in 1984 the Institute of Hearing Research issued a report on 49 discos covering some 4000 young people which showed a hearing loss of .025% at the close of merely one period of attendance. Around some 10% of these young people were open to noise exposure at their work, and a further 10% were at risk from attendance at pop concerts.

In an announcement of a crackdown on noise in work places the Health & Safety Executive indicated that they were also very concerned over the possible hearing damage from leisure activities. In fact the word 'Sociascusis' is now being used to describe any hearing loss related to recreational noise.

## THE EFFECT OF DRUGS

For a number of reasons, this is a difficult area. Much research has yet to be done in the field of drugs relating to tinnitus. The onset of tinnitus can well occur whilst a patient is taking a certain drug but without that particular drug being responsible.

Aspirin, the most commonly used salicylate, is notorious

for its effect on tinnitus, and certainly exacerbates the condition. It usually also induces a hearing loss right across the frequency, but in a few cases the higher frequencies are more strongly acted upon. The hearing loss usually returns to normal after 24 to 72 hours. It has been reported that the tinnitus precedes the hearing loss on the taking of aspirin and diminishes more quickly than the hearing loss itself.

Quinine, and some of the other medications used for the treatment of malaria, are well known in causing temporary hearing loss and tinnitus. The tinnitus so induced is noted before the hearing loss occurs, such hearing loss being of high frequency. Indeed, many experts believe that in persons sensitive to the action of quinine the small amount of this which is contained in the normal 'gin-and-it' is sufficient to induce tinnitus.

## EAR WAX

A further source of tinnitus is believed to be that of wax in the ear. It is not thought that the actual blocking of the ear canal is the cause but that some of the wax has become attached to the tympanic membrane or ear drum. However, others are of the opinion that the existence of wax in the ear canal reduces the volume of external noise, thus revealing an already existing tinnitus.

## EMOTIONAL CHANGES

It has been suggested that an irritation along the organ of Corti can cause a discharge over some of the main auditory fibres in the hearing mechanism and thus bring about a 'narrow band' type of tinnitus. It is also said that any strong emotional changes can cause alterations of the fluids within the inner-ear which could in turn cause sensations of sound within the hearing mechanism. Another theory is that sensory epilepsy within the hearing could well interrupt this mechanism and cause tinnitus to arise from that region.

## EXERCISE

Most people find a definite relation between their tinnitus and circulation in the inner ear, the reason being that the tinnitus increases with exercise because the blood flow is increased.

## HARDENING OF THE ARTERIES

It has been stated in some quarters that tinnitus is connected with hardening of the arteries, but this is very doubtful. Certainly tinnitus is common in people of the older age groups and can co-exist with hardening of the arteries, but there is no evidence that this is a direct result of this condition.

## MÉNIÈRES DISEASE

This complaint usually produces three main symptoms – vertigo, loss of hearing and tinnitus.

The dizziness or vertigo is obviously caused by the body's balance mechanism in the inner ear becoming swollen. Usually this affects only one ear, although in some cases both ears can be affected. The symptoms include vomiting, tinnitus, and in some cases a flickering of the eyes. Attacks alternate, some are mild, some severe. It is a condition that is believed to only affect humans and is more frequent among white people than in coloured.

This is a disease regarded as being in some way associated with industry and urbanisation. The hearing loss, which is usually in the lower frequencies, occurs mostly in one ear in which there is a feeling of pressure or fullness. A hearing loss of up to 30 dB is usual, and this is liable to fluctuation varying with the attacks of vertigo. Gradually this hearing loss increases with time.

Another symptom of this disease can be 'recruitment' an exaggerated sensation of hearing following any increase in the intensity of sound, and this symptom has already been discussed.

With the impairment of hearing in Ménière's Disease normally in the low frequency, the associated tinnitus is in the low frequency range also, so that the patient complains of a low pitched sound as the roaring of wind, or a low buzzing sound. In the efforts that have been made to match sounds of tinnitus caused by this disease it has been reported that the sounds heard are below 1000hz but it is stressed that by no means are these sounds musical or even tonal.

For some time now many treatments have been advocated in efforts to combat this disease, ranging from surgical intervention mainly in attempting to alleviate the vertigo symptoms and ignoring the hearing loss (some surgical procedures are destructive), to drug therapy. This treatment has included reducing sodium in the patient's diet, the prescribing of diuretics to increase the flow of urine, vasodilators which cause widening of the lumen of blood vessels, histamines, tranquillizers, and antihistamines.

The most effective treatment discovered so far in the drug field has been Betahistine Hydrochloride known as Serc which is of benefit in reducing the dizziness, deafness, and consequent tinnitus found in this disease. Serc has not been found of help in other forms of tinnitus, unfortunately.

The one fortunate piece of news that can be given to anyone suffering from Ménière's Disease is that the condition often goes into remission for long periods of time. However the assertion made by some that it 'burns itself out' is a little misleading.


## PERSONAL CASSETTE PLAYERS (P.C.P's)

These easily portable tape machines used with headphones have become extremely popular with young people, allowing them to listen to what amounts to a realistically high level of sound as though actually 'in the room', but many articles have been published warning people of the dangers of hearing loss by their constant use. However some factual information is badly needed to really bring the message home – such as details of listening levels, listening habits, types of music most popular, and length of time used.

The R.N.I.D. Scientific & Technical Department has already studied a number of tests on P.C.P.s and find the maximum sound levels at around 117 dB(A) with normal listening levels at 95 dB(A) with variations of some 15 decibels either way. However, there are many other facts to be taken into consideration, and they feel it too early to draw any firm conclusions from the study at the moment.

Many users of hearing aids and hearing attachments to radios or TVs report that their tinnitus appears to be much worse immediately after such use, as it does with the use of headphones.

## PHANTOM HEARING

It will be obvious that any damage to the nerves of the inner ear – which is the usual cause of hearing loss – means that fewer sound impulses are being sent out to the brain via the hearing nerves. In such a situation it is said that the hearing nerves in the absence of normal outside stimulation may begin to create their own stimulation. The result is tinnitus. This effect is somewhat similar to the pain that some people can feel in an amputated limb.

## PRE-MENSTRUAL TENSION

*Letter:* Is it possible that pre-menstrual tension can aggravate tinnitus? My tinnitus always seems worse at this time.
*Reply:* Pre-menstrual tension certainly aggravates some forms of tinnitus, and if there is any evidence of Ménières-like conditions where there is an increased pressure in the inner ear, then this may be due to fluid retention. Any tension or anxiety also makes a subjective symptom worse, and tinnitus is no exception.

## SPORTING GUNS

An accepted cause of tinnitus is the use of sporting guns or rifles or any involvement with sudden loud noise without the use of ear protection. It is very wrong to engage in any of these activities without protecting one's ears the whole time.

> *Letter:* I worked in a noisy engine testing department for 20 years and although I used some ear protection for most of that time there were no ear protectors in the 1950s and now that I have left that job I still have this constant whistling in one ear and I have it for every waking minute of the day and I have been driven nearly insane at times. . . . I have seriously considered having my hearing destroyed in the offending ear by surgery, but have been advised against this.

> *Letter:* I sometimes wonder about the cause of my tinnitus. Was it being on the 12-pounder gun platform without plugs? On the other hand the noise is similar to the temporary one I had in 1935–40 at the beginning of each tour in West Africa at the resumption of taking quinine each day.
> *Reply:* It is quite possible that your tinnitus does relate to your noise exposure with guns. It is not so much a permanent record of the noise to which you were exposed, but noise generated by the inner ear which has been directly damaged by the sound. Often the tinnitus so produced does not come on for many years after the event.

## DOES SYRINGING CAUSE TINNITUS?

It is now generally accepted that in certain cases syringing of the ears can precipitate tinnitus through causing changes of pressure in the external and middle ear. But this is not thought to be the sole cause by any means. Although there is certainly some link, the situation would be far worse with no means of removing wax, for the wax itself can cause tinnitus in some cases.

Much of the syringing that is at present being undertaken could be avoided if people would abstain from poking things into their ears believing this to be necessary in order to keep their ears clean. Our ears have their own automatic cleansing mechanism, and are best left alone in this respect.

Many patients have reported to the B.T.A. that their tinnitus started immediately following the syringing of their ears, but experts believe that although syringing may well sometimes be the initiating factor in the onset of the condition, these people's ears were susceptible to the condition from the outset, and it would only be a matter of time before tinnitus occurred anyway.

It is not possible to perforate a healthy ear drum with water, although there have been some cases in which the tip of the syringe has perforated the ear drum – the consequences of which have been disastrous. On the other side of the coin it must be remembered that this method of safely removing wax from the ears has resulted in the restoration of hearing to thousands of people.

*Letter:* During a routine medical examination it was recommended that my ears be syringed to remove a considerable accumulation of wax. This was duly carried out, but I have become a sufferer from tinnitus ever since.

## TELEPHONES

Since the left ear is more usually affected than the right it has been suggested that since one uses the left hand in order to leave the right hand free for writing when telephoning, the constant use of the telephone over a long period might eventually cause loss of hearing and tinnitus in the left ear.

## TOBACCO, ALCOHOL, CAFFEINE, etc.

A few experts are of the strong opinion that tobacco is a common cause of tinnitus, but this assertion has not yet been proved in any way. Another cause is said to be caffeine, but little information is available on any research having been made in this connection.

Alcohol is said by some to be a prime culprit; by others an excellent treatment! From the reports available on this particular issue it would seem that an excess of alcohol can certainly cause tinnitus in *some* people, whereas others find small amounts helpful in controlling the symptom, but perhaps in these cases the relaxing effect of the alcohol is the most important feature.

It is said that cocaine and marijuana exacerbate tinnitus, but no detailed information on dosage or quantities appears to be available. Certain oral contraceptives are certainly known to produce tinnitus and hearing loss, probably due to their effect on the blood vessels.

## TRIGGERS

*Letter:* My very high pitched whistle varies from moderate to intolerable within a quarter of an hour and now takes a day or more to fade again. Noises of many kinds bring on my severe attacks, my best defence being to seek quiet environments and to use ear plugs.

Two particular items of modern living trigger a sharp increase in tinnitus level in both ears. The first is the proximity of a 625 line television set with or without the sound. The 15.625 Hz whistle, which I cannot hear, seems to be the culprit. My tinnitus, which is constant in pitch, seems to consist of two notes, this 15 KHz frequency and the octave below at which frequency I have considerable hearing loss (7500 Hz).

The other trigger is almost all cars. In both cases the sound pressure levels are at frequencies I cannot hear but can detect as a feeling of numbness and pressure followed by the tinnitus increasing in volume, and giddy sensations and the like. I find that a car full of people affects me much less than one in which I am driving alone. Recent models which use thin metal body panels have a much worse effect on me. I suspect that panel and exhaust resonances are not carried out at these low frequencies because they are not audible.

Perhaps sound pressure levels above the levels considered damaging would be revealed by such tests if they were carried out!

*Reply:* The tinnitus that you experience which is triggered by certain sounds is encountered fairly commonly in our practice, but is nevertheless a rather particular kind of tinnitus, and your comments would not apply to the majority of tinnitus sufferers. The ear is largely insensitive to frequencies below 15Hz but there has been some interesting work done by Dr Bryan at Salford University on low frequency hearing, and it seems that some people are particularly sensitive to these frequencies.

## TUMOURS

The onset of tinnitus in one ear can be a symptom of a small tumour affecting the eighth nerve. Other symptoms that can follow are dizziness and the loss of high frequency sounds. Fortunately most of such tumours are non-malignant. The usual cause of the deafness and tinnitus in such cases is the compression of other tissues. However, let it be said that hearing loss in one ear and the arrival of tinnitus *in no way* indicates for certain that one has an eighth-nerve tumour.

## VISUAL DISPLAY UNITS

*Letter:*  I have had tinnitus for approximately twelve months and it seemed to occur after working for six months with a particular sort of visual display unit which emitted an audible frequency of around 15.6 KHz. Unfortunately, I am the only person in the office that has sufficiently sensitive hearing to detect this frequency, and no other person has been affected. I have been through the N.H.S. mill of circulatory drugs, and none have been remotely effective. It would be of great interest to myself if you could confirm or deny the obvious conclusion that hearing this frequency for eight hours a day over a six months period would definitely cause the tinnitus.
*Reply:*  I think it unlikely that the high frequency sound that you have been exposed to is of sufficient intensity to have caused the tinnitus. It is quite common, however, for many people in an office not to be able to hear frequencies around 15 KHz.

## CAN TINNITUS BE INHERITED?

The subject has been raised as to whether there is a higher incidence of ear problems in the families of those who suffer from tinnitus. There is no obvious pattern of such inheritance although one consultant has found 35% of tinnitus sufferers had a family history of either deafness or tinnitus.

# IV

# The Treatment of Tinnitus

## NO SINGLE REMEDY

Hitherto specialists have been able to offer very little real hope to sufferers, but fortunately with the recent increased interest in the condition, and the activities of the British Tinnitus Association in particular, the prospect is rapidly changing with at least some palliative reliefs now available. Considerable advances have recently been made in the science of masking, and this has become one of the most popular and successful treatments to date.

As for drugs, unfortunately each drug which has the capacity to help tinnitus has its own unpleasant side effects which prevent universal acceptance and usage. At present those drugs closely related to lidocaine, carbamazepine and sodium amylobarbitone are being closely studied in this connection.

Any helpful treatment is naturally welcomed by sufferers even if it is merely palliative, though of course *complete cure* is the paradise they seek; but since there are so many origins and causes of tinnitus it is fairly evident that no single remedy will be discovered.

## HEARING AIDS & HEARING LOSS

At present there appears to be increasing evidence that both hearing aids and maskers (and this would include hearing instruments which are a combination of both) *can* create a risk to hearing, and it seems possible that the wearing of aids, although relieving the immediate problem may have the ultimate effect over a period of time of causing further hearing loss.

However, as things stand at present, with no acceptable alternative, it is very unlikely that this would dissuade specialists from prescribing such aids, or make hard-of-hearing patients willing to relinquish them, in precisely the same way as some drugs are still continued although their long term effects are all too well known.

To many sufferers tinnitus is a debilitating condition, completely spoiling the quality of life for them, and in a number of cases causing them to become suicidal. One specialist alone has reported that four of his patients have taken their own lives. Such people would doubtless regard a further hearing loss that might occur in the longer term a fair price to pay for any relief obtained.

For tinnitus sufferers at present *low level* masking and aiding is certainly the safer road until more is known on levels of amplification gained from the experience of wearers of aids and maskers. Fortunately now after many years of being passed over by the medical profession because so little was known on the subject, tinnitus is becoming an acknowledged area of research, and regarded with increasing importance.


## TINNITUS & HEARING LOSS

It is fairly usual for those people with tinnitus to also have a certain degree of hearing loss. However, it is not impossible for people to experience tinnitus without any perceivable hearing loss. Our hearing covers a wide band of frequencies and some sufferers from tinnitus regarded as having normal hearing may be found to have actually lost some hearing but only in the untested area above 8 kHz. This is supported somewhat by the widely held view that tinnitus is the fore-runner of hearing loss.


## DIAGNOSING THE CAUSE

Since tinnitus is not a disease in itself, but a symptom of many causes and diseases, only some of which are known, it is surely only logical that the first thing that should be done is to endeavour to diagnose the cause and treat this, rather than immediately turn to maskers, hearing aids, drugs, and the like.

Admittedly in the light of present knowledge certain causes of tinnitus cannot be treated, but it is still the duty of any physician to try to establish the cause, in case treatment *is* possible.

Let us look at the matter in this light. The immediate adoption of maskers, hearing aids and treatment by drugs, all of which have but a palliative effect, may well be hiding signs of a serious problem. Such instances are admittedly rare, but sufferers from tinnitus, in addition to the usual audiological tests, should also have a complete medical examination slanted towards those problems recognised as likely to be the underlying causes of their difficulties.

Take but two examples: if blood pressure is the cause of the tinnitus, or if kidney function is the cause (it is recognised that the functions of ear and kidney are somewhat similar) – then tinnitus maskers and so on are hardly the right treatment.

Several experts recommend that tinnitus sufferers should always receive a medical examination including tests for any infection of the head, neck, and teeth, tests for signs of diabetes, migraine, or for a number of other causes. Yet how often is this done?

# V

# Tinnitus Maskers

Tinnitus sufferers are obtaining various degrees of relief by the use of the modern tinnitus masker. This device produces a band of noise of sufficient frequency content and intensity to mask the noise of the tinnitus. Most maskers produce a broad frequency hissing sound. Many find a masker of special use at night time when the tinnitus is often at its worst with environmental noise at its lowest level. It is without doubt a very significant contribution to the control of tinnitus, but unfortunately it is not a *cure*.

Just as there are various kinds of tinnitus, so there are different types of masker. For example, many sufferers with considerable hearing loss will find that the normal hearing aid gives little relief from their tinnitus when used alone, but a small masking attachment with a fair range of adjustment fitted to the hearing aid can often prove very helpful. A masker alone can also be fitted of course where there is no appreciable hearing loss, and thus no need for a hearing aid.

It is most essential, however, that any such device should be fitted and adjusted by a properly qualified person, and the wearer given careful instruction in making his or her own adjustments. Even then the fitting must be followed up by regular counselling and checking. Alas, there can still be no guarantee of relief in all cases.

Although in certain patients tinnitus cannot be masked, in others practically any weak noise band has a masking effect, and for such people it is possible that environmental noise itself is sufficient to mask their tinnitus. All this merely goes to accentuate the great variety of causes and degrees of the problem.

*Letter:* Why do the British Tinnitus Association go on and on about maskers? We don't want added noise, we want relief from the noises we already suffer. After all there must be a lot of sufferers who cannot get any benefits from a masker?

*Reply:*    The reason why the B.T.A. go on and on about maskers is that the correct fitting of a tinnitus masker is the only symptomatic treatment that has been found to have a significant effect on tinnitus. In the 1930s people were saying exactly the same thing about nerve deafness as you are now about nerve tinnitus. That is to say that there must be some diet or vitamin or simple solution which will just get rid of it. However, nerve tinnitus, which most of our patients suffer, is a disorder that results from the irreversible degeneration of tiny hair cells in the inner ear. These cells cannot be reborn and do not repair themselves, consequently many people with tinnitus find that it does not go away with the application of simple remedies. In the 1930s the early hearing aids were heralded with the same sort of derision as tinnitus maskers are receiving from many quarters at the present time. However, 50 years on hearing aids have become largely acceptable treatment for the management of nerve deafness. I wonder if it will take as long for maskers to catch on?

*Letter:*    Four years ago I had severe tinnitus and was fortunate enough to see Mr Hazell and his genuine concern and compassion for tinnitus sufferers, in contrast to my own doctor's indifference, made me try masking. To start with I wore the masker only when sitting down and I must admit after two weeks or so I felt it wasn't of much benefit, and taking it on and off seemed to emphasise the fact that something was wrong with me. I then decided to wear it constantly, indoors and out. A miracle! After about nine months it seemed that although the tinnitus was not masked completely, I really no longer 'heard' the sounds . . . if the tinnitus wakes me up during the night I simply put my masker on and soon drift back to sleep . . . I have found peace with my masker and am truly grateful to Mr Hazell and everyone who dedicate their lives to improving the quality of ours.

## DISCOVERING THE SITE OF ORIGIN

It has been found that in certain patients with tinnitus only in the one ear, masking can be effected with various tones and bands of noise applied to the other ear. It is not thought that this is caused by cross-conduction, for the amount of volume necessary to mask the tinnitus is in many cases less when applied to the non-tinnitus ear than it is when applied to the ear producing the tinnitus.

The explanation of this so-called 'contralateral masking' is that it produces a reduction of tinnitus signal strength at source. It is also thought that such masking effects itself at some point at which the information coming from both ears meets. It is something that certainly needs much further research and the results would be especially useful to the makers of tinnitus maskers and instruments.

Finding the actual site of the origin of tinnitus would prove a useful breakthrough in many cases, and needs study. It has been discovered that when tonal maskers are used on both ears something between 8 and 15 dB more intensity is needed than with the masking of one ear. This is similar to a phenomenon found in external sound and known as 'masking-level difference'.

## SOUNDS THAT RELIEVE TINNITUS

The beneficial effects of environmental masking of tinnitus have been known from earliest times. The substitution of a pleasant relaxing sound such as music for the sound of an irritating buzz or whine is but a simple example, and one used by many sufferers. Music that is easy on the ear and does not require concentrated listening is probably the most effective, and especially useful in relaxing the listener when engaged in some activity that requires a certain amount of concentration elsewhere. Other sounds that sufferers report as being useful are the sounds of the waves on the shore, wind through the trees, or even just an electric fan. Usually the preference is controlled by the type of tinnitus the person has, whether it be a buzz, a whine, or a whistle or whatever, and at what degree of intensity.

It is strange that some sounds are pleasant to listen to and others highly annoying. Even the same sound under differing circumstances can alter dramatically – music coming from a neighbour's radio can annoy, but tune in the same programme on your own set and all is well. The noise of a slipping chalk irritates us all, but sounds evenly spread across

# Tinnitus Maskers

## (a) Behind the Ear

Chart based on information supplied by Manufacturers/
Importers listed below but please note Tinnitus Maskers
are supplied through hearing aid dispensers
(or tinnitus clinics).

| Manufacturer/ Importer | Country of Origin | Model | Masker or combined masker/hearing aid | Battery type§ | Tone control | Output dB SPL | Price |
|---|---|---|---|---|---|---|---|
| P.C. Werth | (UK) | VTM 1 | masker | SP 675 | yes | 85 | £127 TP |
| P.C. Werth | (UK) | HTM 1 | masker | SP 675 | yes | 84 | £127 TP |
| P.C. Werth | (UK) | Micro | masker | RM 13 | yes | 94 | £165 TP |
| P.C. Werth | (UK) | Micro X | masker | RM 13 | yes | 100 | £165 TP |
| Starkey | (USA) | TM3 | masker | RM 675 | user pre-set | 79/74 | ** |

| Manufacturer | Country | Model | Type | Battery | Control | | Price |
|---|---|---|---|---|---|---|---|
| Starkey | (USA) | TM5 (high frequency) | masker | RM 675 | user pre-set | 41/69 | ** |
| Starkey | (USA) | MA 3 | masker/aid | RM 675 | user pre-set | 79/94 | ** |
| A & M | (UK) | 780 TM | masker | RM 675 | yes | 84 | £126 |
| Bonochord | (Austria) | ARTI | masker | R13 | no | 75 | £309 |
| Bonochord | (Austria) | ARPPTI | masker | R13 | no | 126 | £367 |
| Bonochord | (Austria) | AMTI | masker | R675 | yes | 88 | £188 |
| Bonochord | (Austria) | 116 series A | masker/aid | R675 | yes | 70 | £403 |
| Bonochord | (Austria) | 116 series P | masker/aid | R675 | yes | 90 | £460 |
| Danovox | (Denmark) | Range available | masker/unit | RM 675 | yes | 105 | £300-£380 |

## (b) Bedside

| | | | | | 90/Pillow Free field | |
|---|---|---|---|---|---|---|
| P.C. Werth | (USA) | Sleep-a-Tone | masker | 3X MN 1604 | yes | 90/Pillow Free field | £195 |
| G. Williams | (UK) | Bedside | masker | 1XPP3 | no | 115 | £115 with timer |

## (c) In the ear

| | | | | | | |
|---|---|---|---|---|---|---|
| P.C. Werth | (UK) | EM6TM | masker | RM 13 | yes | variable | £419 |
| Starkey | (USA) | TM1 | masker | RM 13 | yes | 70-107 | ** |
| Starkey | (USA) | MA1 | Masker/aid | RM 13 | no | 70-107 | ** |
| Bonochord | (Austria) | AZTI | masker | R13 | no | 80 | £450 |
| G. Williams | (UK) | Ear Canal | masker | 312 | no | 78 | £51 |
| G. Williams | (UK) | Ear Canal | masker | 312 | yes | 75 | £90 |

# (d) Spectacle

| | | | | Battery§ | | | Price |
|---|---|---|---|---|---|---|---|
| Bonochord | (Austria) | ASTI | Bone Conduction | R675 | no | – | £495 |
| Bonochord | (Austria) | ALTI | Air Conduction | R675 | yes | 85 | £427 |

§Battery types refer to those most commonly used but alternatives are available.
** Starkey do not suggest retail prices. TP denotes that the price includes a trial period.
For further information and names and addresses of retailers apply direct to the manufacturers/importers:

P.C. Werth Ltd.,
Audiology House,
45 Nightingale Lane,
London SW12 8SP
(Tel: 01-675 5151)

G. Williams Hearing Aid Services
The Old Mill,
23 Greenwich High Road,
Greenwich, London SE10 8JL
(Tel: 01-692 0302)

Starkey Laboratories Ltd.
Unit 3, Deanway,
Wilmslow Road, Handforth,
Wilmslow, Cheshire SK9 3HW
Tel: Wilmslow (0625) (529223)

A & M Hearing Aids Ltd.,
Faraday Road,
Crawley, Sussex RH10 2LS
(Tel: Crawley (0293) 540471)

Bonochord Hearing Aids Ltd.,
London Road, Riverhead,
Sevenoaks, Kent TN13 2DN
(Tel: Sevenoaks (0732) 459181)

Danavox (GB) Ltd.,
1 Cheyne Walk,
Northampton
(Tel: Northampton (0604) 36351)

the auditory spectrum are generally accepted as being more pleasant. A sound at which the pitch is more or less at the same level and therefore predictive is undoubtedly more distracting and annoying than one of a more changing nature. Those sounds in which the energy is spread over a wider spectrum (i.e. a broad noise band) will always be found to be far less annoying.

From various studies, it does appear that tinnitus sufferers are less upset by annoying sounds than others. Perhaps this can be put down to the fact that they have had to learn to live with an irritating noise for some time and in consequence have become a little more tolerant of this particular annoyance.

## RESIDUAL INHIBITION

The idea has been put forward that possibly those sounds which help in masking tinnitus actually stimulate over a wider area than the tinnitus itself. A surprising outcome of masking is that often the tinnitus is reduced in intensity after the masker has been switched off; in some cases it has been reported that it has disappeared completely. Unfortunately this effect, which is known as residual inhibition, does not last for long, and usually the tinnitus will resume after a few minutes, although there are reports of it disappearing for days, weeks, and sometimes months! It appears that residual inhibition occurs to differing degrees dependent on the type of tinnitus.

Unfortunately the mechanics behind residual inhibition are not fully understood yet and much further research is needed in this field, which could perhaps have the effect of improving the design of maskers.

The best advice that can be given at present is that users of maskers should tune the level of intensity to the very lowest level at which it masks their tinnitus.

## SOUND MATCHING

Much further research is also badly needed concerning the

actual sounds heard by sufferers of tinnitus. Mere vocal description is really very inadequate. Ten years ago one researcher produced recorded sounds based on the descriptions of tinnitus given him by his patients. But few of these examples appeared to match precisely what the patients were actually hearing.

An ordinary music synthesizer has been used to try to match up with the sounds heard by various patients, but this takes considerable time, and cannot of course apply to all types of the condition, though where successful it would of course provide an excellent objective method of explanation, far more satisfactory than any verbal description.


## PITCH MATCHING

Some experimenters have used pitch matching tests in order to try to match in actual pitch the sound of a patient's tinnitus against the sound supplied by external means. However, there are several problems here, for many people except trained musicians easily make what is known as 'octave errors' – this is especially likely to occur when in an endeavour to match pitch an ordinary audiometer is used. Another problem that arises with the audiometer is the likelihood of the tinnitus being grossly under-estimated, especially with high frequency tinnitus. Most audiometers do not range above 8kHz thus a patient with for example a 12kHz high pitch tinnitus would find it impossible to match and would probably settle for a 6kHz tone. Again, tinnitus itself often fluctuates in pitch (2 to 5 kHz difference has been found over different sessions). So great a fluctuation does not seem to be a common experience, but it is certainly a feature that should be known by those who design tinnitus maskers and instruments.

# VI

# Drugs on Trial for the Treatment of Tinnitus

Medication with drugs for the relief of tinnitus has not so far proved very successful, the effect of all drugs on the condition, where there is any effect, being essentially dose-related. Unfortunately for most tinnitus sufferers to obtain any effect at all the dose is usually at least that at which toxic side effects occur. This factor has thus limited the use of drugs dramatically in this particular field, for present day drugs are very powerful and can sometimes produce quite dangerous side-effects. It is of course possible to minimise such side-effects by only gradually increasing the dosage (a method that has been used with some success in New Zealand), but of course drugs should never be used at all except under the strictest medical supervision, and even then the advantages must be strongly weighed against the disadvantages.

Many of the drugs under trial for tinnitus are medically known as 'membrane stabilisers' which appear to have a calming effect on the excitability of nerve cells, causing a nerve to require a stronger stimulus for a message to be passed along it. It also increases the length of the 'refractory period' i.e. the length of time before the nerve is capable of reacting again.

The use of drugs in the area of tinnitus suppression is particularly difficult, for tinnitus, as we have seen, is not a disease but a symptom with very many different causes, and until continued research enables the actual site causing the tinnitus to be definitely identified then treatment is of necessity very much a matter of trial and error. Coupled to this is the fact that those drugs known as 'membrane stabilisers', like all other drugs, have certain side-effects.

If only more funding were available for research so much

more could be done in the exploration of drug treatments for tinnitus: for example the effects of drugs could be monitored by using such modern techniques as transtympanic electro-cochieography, a system capable of monitoring any changes taking place in the cochlea and cochlea nerve.

As things stand at present researchers are obliged to rely mainly on the reports of patients as to whether or not their tinnitus has improved under any treatment – it should be possible for all such tests to be assessed far more objectively than this.

## CARBAMAZEPINE (Tegretol)

This is a mild antidepressant and anticonvulsant drug taken orally and has been used on the continent for the treatment of epilepsy. Unfortunately it has a wide variety of side effects. In experiments with this drug some patients have been found to benefit from it, who obtained only small relief from lidocaine; yet other patients who obtained some excellent results from lidocaine had but little relief from carba-mazepine, which is some indication of the difficulties that surround research in this field. In view of its side effects and the fact that it is very poorly tolerated by many, carba-mazepine has obviously very limited use in the general treatment of tinnitus, at least until further research finds solutions to the difficulties.

## LIDOCAINE (Lignocaine) (Xlocaine)

An injection of this drug has been found to have a short term effect on tinnitus and thus its possibilities are being researched.

In one study 78 sufferers with severe tinnitus were treated. Before the injection of lidocaine the standard audiological examination was given, and following the injection the patients requested to show any improvement in their tinnitus by placing a mark on a 100mm line. It is assumed that this was done within a few minutes of the injection.

In this particular study 35% of the sufferers found the tinnitus completely gone, 28% reported it to be slightly less intense, and 26% said they found no lessening whatever of the condition. Interestingly, the 'reliefs' varied from between ten minutes up to three whole days. With some of those finding relief there was also an improvement in their hearing, but this was not felt to be very important since it is usual for reports of improvements in hearing to be made following any tests of drugs on tinnitus.

Another interesting study of the effect of this drug was made in 1980 when 592 sufferers from fairly severe tinnitus were injected with lidocaine and one minute after the injection asked to estimate their relief in percentages. The sufferers were divided into two groups – those unilaterally affected, and those with the condition in both ears. Curiously, more of the latter reported relief than did those unilaterally afflicted. Yet 6% with bilateral affliction had no relief at all; as did 27% of those with unilateral tinnitus. This differing result in the use of lidocaine is felt to have considerable importance for future research.

## NIACIN

Although this drug has been used with a certain amount of success in the treatment of Ménière's Disease and patients have reported a lessening of the intensity of their tinnitus, it can in no way be regarded as a general treatment for tinnitus itself.

## PHENYTOIN SODIUM (Dilantin) (Epanutin)

This is a drug taken orally, and is very similar in its action to carbamazepine, although it has been found to be very much less effective in the treatment of tinnitus. It also has a particularly high incidence of side effects.

## PRIMIDONE (Mysoline)

Primidone is an anticonvulsant and a study of its effects on tinnitus was undertaken as far back as 1980. The published result showed that 27% of the patients treated felt they had between 80% and 100% relief from tinnitus; there were however reports of considerable side effects.

## SODIUM AMYLOBARBITONE

There appears to be evidence that this drug effectively diminishes the disturbance caused by tinnitus, although its use is somewhat limited owing to the fact that liver damage can result. However, a very promising outcome of one experiment was that six weeks after cessation of the drug four subjects who initially reported that their tinnitus had been abolished were still found to be free of it, and there were no significant alterations in the conditions reported by other subjects of the experiment at the close of treatment. The drug has been used for many years in the treatment of epilepsy but owing to the ease with which patients can become addicted and with the introduction of more efficient drugs for sedation, there currently exists a strong recommendation for banning the drugs of this particular group.

## SODIUM FLUORIDE

This is known to have an effect on the cochlea capsule. Its administration does not in any way improve hearing loss but it does have an effect on tinnitus and vertigo.

## SODIUM VALPROATE (Depakene) (Epilim) (Ergenyl)

Here is a drug which has been found to reduce tinnitus in approximately the same proportion of subjects as carbamazepine, although the amount of relief from it has been found to be a little less than with the use of carbamazepine, but in compensation its side effects are also less.


## TOCAINIDE HYDROCHLORIDE (Tocard)

Another drug that has been tried against tinnitus. In one study patients were injected at intervals of six hours, four times a day. Some of the group were given exactly the same amount of tocainide or a placebo every other six hour interval. Some were merely given a placebo four times a day.

Of the 56 sufferers included in the experiment 11 of these withdrew due to reported side effects (yet two of these had received only the placebo). An hour and a half following the final dose those taking part were asked to judge the degree of relief from their tinnitus. The result was that between 40% and 100% relief was reported by 41% of those who had received two doses a day, and 7% of those who had merely received a placebo.


## OTHER DRUGS

Some other drugs that have been tried in the treatment of tinnitus include naftidrofuryl, lorcainide, bupivacaine, arlidin, chlortrimeton and nortriptyline . . . (There must surely exist an army of boffins dreaming up new names for drugs!)

The popular valium (diazepam) has been fairly frequently prescribed for tinnitus and its accompanying depression, but experts report there is absolutely no evidence that it has any value in the reduction of tinnitus, and can in actual fact exacerbate a patient's condition.

Maxilitine has been tried. This is a drug closely related to lidocaine and can be administered orally; however its effects have been more than disappointing.

*Letter:* I feel desperate for some kind of relief from the tinnitus which I have had for the past six years. I have consulted two specialists and numerous hospitals but the tinnitus just seems to get worse, and I can see no future in life at all. My own doctor prescribed librium tablets but these are of little help. If there are any tablets or anything that can give me relief from this illness I would be grateful to hear from you.

*Reply:*   Librium and other nerve tablets do not usually do much to change the tinnitus itself although they can help to allay the attendant anxiety. There *are* some tablets and drugs which *do* help slightly in tinnitus, and these are being investigated in drug trials at present.

*Letter:*   Recently in a German newspaper the question came from a tinnitus sufferer and the answer was given by a Dr von Miendorf that 'there is now a new medicine from Belgium called Melopal with ingredients Betahistin. Tinnitus goes away' – is this medicine available in this country?

*Reply:*   The drug you mention, Betahistine is available in this country and is called Serc. It is a very effective treatment for Ménière's Disease, one of the symptoms of which is tinnitus. When it is effective in Ménière's Disease the tinnitus goes away. The disease is a relatively rare condition, and if you do not have it but have tinnitus for one or other of many other reasons Serc will do you no good at all.

*Letter:*   I was prescribed Ledefen for arthritis . . . but my tinnitus has suddenly become very much worse. . . Is there any drug which will relieve me and not cause tinnitus?

*Reply:*   All drugs taken for rheumatism may cause tinnitus in susceptible people. However, the tinnitus is always related to the dose taken, and should go away when you stop taking the drug. If it does not go away . . . then it is most probably not related to the drug therapy at all. As tinnitus and arthritis are both so common it is not unusual for the two to coexist.

*Letter:*   I was interested to read in your letters column that Tegretol has side effects, and as this directly concerns me I would like to know more about these side effects. It gives me extreme drowsiness, and I would like to know if the bad headaches, heaviness above the eyes and forehead, and extreme unbalance especially in the dark, are connected?

*Reply:*   All the symptoms you describe could be due to the Tegretol. One of the problems with this drug is that it is very poorly tolerated by some people. This is a great pity, because it is so effective in reducing tinnitus levels.

*Letter:*   I have noted readers' letters who find alcohol helps their tinnitus, and you recommend a drug called nicotinic acid in these cases. I too find whisky helps my tinnitus. Does this mean the nicotinic acid will 'definitely' help if alcohol helps? Can you tell me what strength of tablet is recommended and how often should one take a dosage?

*Reply:* I'm afraid the answer is not 'definitely'. Only a small proportion of people who are helped by alcohol find nicotinic acid any good. The prescription is nicotinic acid 50mg three times a day, increasing by 50mg three times a day until flushing occurs.

*Letter:* Tinnitus struck me quite suddenly . . . my doctor sent me to see a specialist at an ENT clinic . . . he gave me a prescription for Tegretol which I have been taking ever since. However, just lately I find that at times I must increase the dosage. I do not wish to go on taking Tegretol for the rest of my life as the prescriptions cost so much.

*Reply:* You are one of the very few people who are helped by this drug. I have just answered a pile of letters from people desperate for the name of a drug which will relieve their tinnitus, although I know that drugs are most unlikely to do this. Incidentally, if you are likely to go on taking Tegretol for a long time, there are schemes whereby you can pay less than the cost of a prescription each time. A properly fitted tinnitus masker might mean that you could stop taking the drugs altogether.

*Letter:* Knowing that as yet there is no known cure for tinnitus and that different kinds of drugs have been tried by sufferers, what about the new wonder drug Interferon?

*Reply:* Interferon is a drug which activates the immunological response of the body, and helps it to fight against things like viruses and cancer cells which are then treated as foreign material. We do not think it would have any place in the treatment of tinnitus which is neither a cancer nor an infection.

*Letter:* I am being treated in hospital for traces of TB. Since 1974 I have suffered from partial deafness and tinnitus. I am naturally anxious that this condition will not be aggravated by any drug treatment . . . will any of the drugs used for TB have adverse effects?

*Reply:* You are right in thinking that the drugs used for the treatment of tuberculosis can cause tinnitus and deafness. This is especially true if Streptomycin injections are being given. It is most important that whilst you are having treatment your hearing should be measured at weekly intervals on an audiometer including frequencies up to 8 kHz and preferably above this if the instrument is capable of it. The first sign of any deterioration in the high frequencies should indicate to those concerned that further Streptomycin therapy should only be continued if there is no alternative treatment available. In view of your history it would be a good idea if treatment were to be considered with one of the alternative drugs such as Rifampacin.

*Letter:* I am enclosing a cutting from a Canadian newspaper . . .

which states that Tocaine Hydrocholoride is now judged to be an acceptable cure for tinnitus.

*Reply:* Unfortunately this is just a piece of irresponsible journalism. The Emmett and Shea paper to which the Canadian newspaper refers included an uncontrolled trial of tocainide in a very high dose which *did* have a very dramatic effect in six patients. However, Emmett himself is now convinced that this is not the solution to the problem and we have all come across so many patients who have had severe side effects from this drug. Five separate drug trials (double blind control crossover) have been performed in this country, two of them on tocainide hydrocholoride and there is absolutely no evidence that it will help the majority of tinnitus sufferers. However, there are occasional 'responders' and what we need is a way of sorting these from the others.

*Letter:* Whilst on a course of calcium gluconate tablets, the volume and frequency of tinnitus has been reduced almost to nil. I have advised my doctor and the hearing aid service about this, and thought you might be interested.

*Reply:* I am very interested to hear about your experience with calcium gluconate. Although this will probably only help a small proportion of people with tinnitus, I have always thought that some of these more simple compounds ought to have an effect on some patients. The difficulty is that properly controlled trials on all these different substances would take more time than we have available at present.

*Letter:* I see a specialist regularly at a good ENT department and I am constantly reminded by him that there is no treatment for my quite severe tinnitus, but in your reply to a reader's letter you mentioned a drug Tonocard. Are these drugs unknown to outside doctors and ENT specialists? Why should they not be offered?

*Reply:* The first treatment for tinnitus is the fitting of the correct tinnitus masking instrument. When all types have been tried to no avail (this can often take six months) then it is worth trying the drugs in this group. However, many of these have horrendous side-effects and patients have often been made more ill than they were before. This is why they are not to be dished out like sweeties.

Unfortunately, only at those centres where there is a specialist with an interest in tinnitus do you find anything but the attitude that 'nothing can be done and you have to go away and live with it'. It is not a matter of ignorance, it is a matter of disinterest. We are doing what we can to change it.

# VII

# Other Sources of Help

In the absence of any very real help from orthodox quarters, apart from masking, it is only natural that sufferers should wish to explore the possibilities of any other likely sources.

## ACUPUNCTURE

This method of treating illness, by inserting the tips of silver alloy or stainless steel needles into certain parts of the patient's skin and vibrating them, has been explored for the possible relief of tinnitus.

The technique, which was practised in China over 4500 years ago, is very popular today, not only in this country, but is being used increasingly in conjunction with orthodox medicine in North America, Western Europe, Japan, Russia and other countries. A constantly increasing number of medical practitioners are now adding acupuncture to their other skills.

However, unfortunately as regards tinnitus there is little evidence that acupuncture can be of help. The most that reports indicate is that it can be of help in early cases, but one can discover no supportive evidence of this. In a recently controlled trial of acupuncture it was found to be no better than random needle insertion so far as the relief of tinnitus was concerned.

*Letter:* My tinnitus which started a few years ago appears to be worsening slowly. I have received some help from mineral therapy and the identification of a food allergy. Do you think acupuncture would help me?
*Reply:* We have received thousands of letters relating to acupuncture and tinnitus but I am afraid we have had no good reports. There is no reason why tinnitus should respond to

acupuncture despite the claims of the acupuncturists. Our evidence seems to be to the contrary.

*Letter:* I have often read questions asking if acupuncture helps relieve tinnitus at all. I have had almost £300 worth of treatment and it has not made any difference whatsoever. That money was just wasted.

*Letter:* I am twenty nine years old and have suffered from tinnitus for about nine years. I am also very deaf, having lost almost all hearing in one ear and with considerable hearing loss in the other. I have suffered from severe depression and acute anxiety for the same length of time (cause or effect one wonders?) but have now found relief with a series of acupuncture treatments.
   Up to date the tinnitus has not decreased at all, but I seem to have been 'desensitised' and it does not bother me as much. I am less irritable, more relaxed, sleep better and generally enjoy a happier and more healthy life. Perhaps other readers have had similar success with acupuncture?
*Reply:* I think your experience with acupuncture is the best we can expect. As you say your tinnitus has not decreased but your attitude to it has changed and you are less irritable and able to sleep better. That is what we find with most of these treatments, including biofeedback. The fact that you can cope better with troublesome tinnitus can make all the difference.

## BIOFEEDBACK

This is a technique that has been in use by doctors since the 1960s and is used more especially in the treatment of migraine, insomnia and circulatory problems. It is a technique in which the patient monitors bodily responses of which he or she would not otherwise be conscious, and then endeavours to control them through relaxation, breathing exercises, or other disciplines such as Yoga.

The responses thus monitored include skin and muscle tension, various brain rhythms and so on. It has been proved that patients are able to control the 'alpha rhythms' produced by the brain usually in connection with feelings of relaxation, and this makes it a hopeful candidate for the tinnitus sufferer.

Biofeedback is a long term process and needs determination and patience in a training regime utilising electronic equipment to help the patient control blood pressure and anxiety states, and reports of a certain degree of success in this method for the relief of tinnitus have come from New Zealand.

John and Linda House of Los Angeles also report that in a recent study of biofeedback on tinnitus sufferers eight out of ten derived some improvement. Clarke of Alabama has likewise reported success in biofeedback for the condition, but in the case of two of his patients who were on long term therapy it had no effect at all.

Recent research in America has shown that biofeedback is certainly helpful in reducing the anxiety and tension connected with tinnitus, and in some cases has been found to actually reduce the tinnitus.

The body functions usually monitored are heart-rate, blood pressure, skin resistance, and sometimes the alpha-rhythms of the EEG (the electro-encephalogram.) The idea is to learn to control such functions by one's own conscious effort and this usually results in the production of profound relaxation, especially in those patients who suffer from tension. However, this can only be achieved over quite a time, and by using expensive equipment. Even so, only isolated reports of tinnitus improvement following this type of treatment have come to hand.

It certainly does appear that the success of biofeedback is directly related to the patient's own personality, and thus those who most need the help are unfortunately all too often not good at achieving it. The attitude of mind required to benefit from biofeedback is in some ways very similar to that required for the success of yoga.

The aim is to so condition a patient that the induced pattern becomes ingrained and the equipment then unnecessary. A number of these machines can now be purchased on the open market, but it is advisable to seek medical advice before buying, since some, such as the EEG, should only be used under qualified instruction.

Such treatments as hypnosis and biofeedback may well have a beneficial influence on tinnitus in much the same way as stress and depression can have a harmful influence. Hypnosis and self-hypnosis that can control symptoms of stress and produce genuine relaxation can be of nothing but benefit to anyone suffering from tinnitus.

*Letter:* My wife has severe tinnitus . . . she has tried a masker and ordinary hearing aids. The specialist told her these would be of no use to her as she has dead cells which will not regenerate. Numerous pills have not helped her in any way. She has threatened to take her life and is very depressed and cries a lot. We have heard of biofeedback but do not know what this is. Is there a chance of the tinnitus getting less, remaining the same, or getting worse? The doctor told her that nerve cutting would make tinnitus worse. We had looked forward to our retirement but this has now ruined our lives.

*Reply:* Biofeedback techniques have been tried extensively in the States and do seem to help some people with tinnitus. They are particularly helpful with anxious tense people as they reduce the amount of sympathetic discharge in the automatic nervous system which governs things like heart rate and sweating. In some cases this may reduce the level of tinnitus. . . . You are quite right in thinking that cutting the nerve of hearing (nerve section) might make the tinnitus worse. It is true that sometimes it *does* abolish the tinnitus, but unfortunately there is no way of knowing whether it is going to make it better or worse before the operation. As a general rule we advise against nerve section, as this may make certain experimental forms of tinnitus suppression (for instance electrical stimulation) impossible to consider. Should these treatments become widely available in the future and you have had your nerve cut, then these methods of treatment would not be available to you.

## DIET

The general concensus of expert opinion indicates that diet itself has little or no effect on tinnitus. Certainly some people are sensitive or allergic to certain items in their diet, but there exists no specific diet for the relief of tinnitus, despite all that has been written on this subject.

The following letters are included solely because it is felt they may be of interest to readers:

*Letter:* I consulted two doctors who identified tinnitus and at various times was prescribed Stemetil tablets, nasal sprays, and had one ear syringed. None of these gave anything more than short term relief.

I also looked at my life pattern and made various futile attempts to vary or improve it by a better balance of exercise and fresh air in an attempt to combat stress and to remove the roaring, droning noises, and the headaches that accompanied them day and night. . . . Then I turned to my diet looking for unnecessary, unhelpful items. I do not drink or smoke and the obvious first choice appeared to be tea of which I was drinking up to seven cups a day. I gave up drinking tea.

The effect was amazing. Within a day or two the headaches and tinnitus had gone and I have enjoyed months of wonderful release from all that noise and extra strain. I am also much happier and feel healthier eating apples or drinking milk or decaffeinated coffee as replacements for the tea. It is not easy to avoid the odd cup on certain social occasions but although I experience occasional background whistling noises the problem is not acute and I feel there is a measure of control at last. I would not presume that this would solve other people's tinnitus problems but dietary factors would appear to have a strong bearing on the complaint. I note that cheese and marmite adversely affect one reader, but they do not in my case.

*Letter:*   Is there anything I am doing, or eating, that makes my tinnitus get louder? It seems to get louder every day – I do not know how much longer I can stand it. Alcohol makes my tinnitus worse. I always understood this should be only temporary, but it seems to make mine permanently worse.

*Reply:*   It is unlikely that anything in your diet is affecting your tinnitus, provided you eat a fairly normal diet. It is also unlikely that your tinnitus is actually getting louder. But you are probably paying more attention to it, listening to it all day for minor changes in pitch and loudness. This of course makes the tinnitus seem far worse and takes over the whole of your consciousness. As far as possible you should try to ignore the sounds that it makes.

It is true that alcohol affects tinnitus. Some people find that it abolishes it, whereas others find that it makes it worse. It just shows how different tinnitus can be from one case to another. Anti-depressant drugs have also been reported as causing tinnitus, although many patients with tinnitus are severely depressed and are very much better while taking anti-depressants.

*Letter:*   I noticed intermittent noises in my ears. I experimented and found that they followed soon after I had eaten peanuts. I was in Nigeria at the time and ate a lot of peanuts. I stopped eating them (or drinking coffee which increased any existing noise) and had months completely free of any noise. One night I had a handful of peanuts – foolishly – and they acted like a switch. The rushing noise has been constant ever since. I have eaten no peanuts until two weeks ago. Within two to three hours the volume increased . . . I don't understand how the peanuts could affect the ears so quickly. Are some parts of them digested faster than others?

*Reply:* I cannot be sure what it is in the peanuts that is causing the tinnitus. I think that it is very likely that there is some other problem in your ears which is responsible, the peanuts simply precipitating the tinnitus. In about 10% of sufferers the tinnitus is exacerbated by things in their diet and I expect you are one of these.

*Letter:* In 'Vitamin C against Cancer' by H.L. Newbold I read: 'For many years I have experienced a ringing in the ears . . . I did not pay much attention to it . . . however the ringing got really loud and became annoying. I began adding and subtracting foods from my diet because symptoms like mine are often caused by food allergies. In spite of these attempts I was unable to reduce the ringing . . . I began adding and subtracting from my mineral-vitamin regime. I experienced no relief . . . I decided to try increasing my intake of bioflavonoids. As if by magic the ringing had all but disappeared within ten minutes after I took half a teaspoonful of bioflavonoids along with my usual dose of vitamin C. The beneficial effect has continued'.

Some research on the effects of these substances seems warranted since they are cheap, harmless, and nothing else works. A possible rationale for the action of bioflavonoids is that they (in conjunction with Vitamin C) strengthen the walls of blood vessels: and vascular deficiencies are sometimes implicated in tinnitus.

*Reply:* Thank you for your interesting letter. Bioflavonoids (Vitamin B preparations) have been used in the treatment of deafness and tinnitus but generally without success.

*Letter:* Somewhere . . . I read about the beneficial effects of garlic upon tinnitus. Since then, about a year ago I have taken garlic in food whenever possible and the noise level of my tinnitus has decreased significantly. Perhaps not too much importance should be attached to this: the noise level may have decreased anyway, the effect may not be permanent, or garlic may only have an effect on some forms of tinnitus. However may it be worthwhile to investigate if there is any substance in garlic which has an effect on tinnitus?

*Reply:* We have many letters about garlic and its beneficial effects. However, as most people put the garlic in the outer ear rather than eating it, I think in this way it has very little effect on the ear itself.

As I have said before in newsletters, substances placed in the outer canal are not generally absorbed at all through intact skin. But garlic taken by mouth permeates the whole body – as we know! It is particularly excreted through the sweat glands and contains a number of active substances. It would certainly do no harm to try it to see if it helps tinnitus, and I would be very interested to hear if it does.

*The Garlic Recipe* (As given in the B.T.A. Newsletter)

Ingredients:
    2 ozs olive or mustard oil
    8 cloves of garlic (peeled)

Method:
    Heat oil and garlic very gently until cloves turn black. Remove pan from heat and allow to cool. Strain and bottle. Use two to three drops in ear daily and when condition improves use once or twice weekly. This remedy should be used in conjunction with eating three or four cloves of garlic in food.

*The Medical Adviser comments:*   We cannot recommend everyone to try this as some people have conditions of the outer or middle ear which make it imperative that they do not put fluid in the ear.
    Garlic has been used as a cure-all throughout the centuries and there must be some scientific explanation for some of these cases, although one is not forthcoming at present.


## HOMOEOPATHY

This is one of several other possibilities of help to which many tinnitus sufferers have turned. With its holistic approach specifically suited to each individual, involving the treatment of the 'whole patient' as opposed to concentration on a single symptom, it certainly appears to be a sensible approach for tinnitus with its many origins. Even a lifting of tension can often lead to a remission of this distressing condition.

Most doctors have no objection to patients trying different possible remedies, and two important features of homoeopathy lie in the fact that the remedies have no side effects whatever and can also be safely taken in conjunction with any other treatment.

Certainly homoeopathic treatment is far preferable to loads of tranquillisers and sleeping pills.

*Letter:* During the management of a community pharmacy, I have had the opportunity to counter prescribe for several individuals suffering from tinnitus. The background and quality varied tremendously, but in each case I chose a homoeopathic remedy specifically suited to the individual's constitution. The results of this 'holistic approach' have been astonishing. In response to treatment each person noted a reduction in noise level and usually a decrease in frequency. This initial change was followed by a lifting of tensions with expressions such as 'I feel so much better in myself'. Treatment over a period of two months in one person resulted in a complete cure of his tinnitus and his underlying depression. I sincerely believe that treating the person as a whole rather than acting against an isolated symptom can lead to remission of tinnitus.

*Reply:* The attitude of treating the whole patient is to be thoroughly applauded, and should apply whenever a symptom, particularly a chronic symptom, is being treated. Unfortunately comments about successful treatment do not amount to a discovery of a cure for tinnitus, which is a symptom of a very wide variety of different disorders. I'm sure that the writer of this letter did not intend this, but unfortunately tinnitus sufferers who read these testimonials often have their hopes falsely raised.

In our experience of following tinnitus sufferers for many years, and studying as scientifically as possible a wide variety of different treatments, we are struck by the close association between depression and tinnitus. In many patients, successful treatment of depression, something that homoeopathy does so well, may result in a level of tinnitus which was previously intolerable becoming quite acceptable or even ignored. It is not helpful to claim that this is a cure of a symptom representing what is probably the result of degenerative change in the auditory system.

It is vital to keep a completely open mind about treatment possibilities particularly when there is no cure. However, for each letter that we receive with claims of successful treatment of tinnitus by medicine or alternative medicine, we receive 200 letters from patients bemoaning the large amounts of money that have been spent only to have their hopes dashed at the end of some course of ineffective therapy. The important message here is that when people feel much better in themselves, or are released from their feelings of depression, then a wide spectrum of symptoms, anxieties, and environmental pressure will seem far less of a problem, and indeed may cease to exist at all. The problem with the depressed person who has tinnitus is that it is often impossible for him or her to see which symptom is chicken and which is egg.

## HYPNOTHERAPY

Although hypnotherapy would appear to be yet another useful area for exploration, it is unfortunate that the information available to date is not only sparse, but is inclined to indicate a rather poor track record.

A certain amount of information on the subject can be gleaned from some hundred or so letters from tinnitus sufferers on this subject written to the British Tinnitus Association, but alas no writer reports any spectacular benefit from hypnosis. For this reason and in order to give broader coverage of this particular possible source of help to the tinnitus sufferer, I am deeply indebted to Mr Hellmut Karle for permission to include his interesting and valuable report of the hypnosis trial for tinnitus carried out at Guys Hospital in 1984 which appears later in this section.

*Letter:* I have severe very high frequency pulsating tinnitus in both ears. Only a sandblaster tends to drown the sound, but even then I can feel it. The only relief I get is first thing in the morning after a good sleep . . . I am driven to bed in the evening to get away from it. I have a tendency to hypertension and have been undergoing drug therapy for years (10 tablets daily) but as far as I know they have no influence on the tinnitus.

There is a noise limit which like pain can become unbearable, if the noise always remained below this limit there would be no problem. The level of noise varies enormously which prevents one getting used to the sound. Has anyone ever tried hypnosis to persuade the brain to ignore such noises?

*Reply:* Obviously your tinnitus is being aggravated by your tendency to anxiety and depression. The tablets you are taking are principally to help you with these as well as your hypertension and would not be expected to have any effect on the tinnitus itself.

Hypnosis has been tried, but does not seem to have any long-lasting beneficial effect.

*Letter:* You recently invited comments from anyone who had experience of hypnotherapy for tinnitus. I have suffered from this condition for a number of years and in 1977 was introduced to a local qualified practitioner. He frankly admitted that he could not guarantee a cure, but in desperation I visited him weekly for five weeks. During that time he taught me how to induce a mild state of self-hypnosis and relaxation. The visits themselves were most helpful in reducing tension and I have returned occasionally for one visit in order to reinforce his treatment.

The tinnitus has not departed but I am able to induce a condition of complete relaxation which has been a source of amazement to my friends. I find this of considerable help, and after even a few minutes I am refreshed and able to cope with my ear noises. I find the technique advantageous at all times and even my dentist has been both amused and surprised how completely my body relaxes before he starts work.

For those who are sceptical or cynical of hypnotherapy and compare it with certain stage performances I would emphasize that at the hands of a competent practitioner there is absolutely nothing to fear.

The short course to which I submitted has been of inestimable value. I stopped taking Valium and other drugs and apart from occasional medication with Nicotinamide – which I have found useful – I do not have to rely on any of the various prophylactics.

## TINNITUS & HYPNOSIS

by

Hellmut Karle B.A., A.B.Ps.S., Consultant Psychologist & Principal Psychologist at Guy's Hospital, London

Until quite recently available literature on the subject of tinnitus contained details of only one minor trial of hypnosis as a likely means of coping with this condition. Last year Nick Marks, Consultant ENT Surgeon, Con Onisiphorou, Senior Technician in ENT and myself carried out a trial of hypnosis on fourteen patients who were well known to the ENT Department at Guy's Hospital. Indeed, many of them had taken part in previous clinical trials in treatments as diverse as acupuncture and anti-convulsant drugs. None of the patients had gained significant relief from any previously tried treatments. To cut a long story short, only one of the patients reported any lessening of noise in his case. This report was not supported by matching tests.

However, five patients reported marked improvements in other aspects of their state. The use of regular sessions of self-hypnosis was felt by them to increase their tolerance of the tinnitus, although there was no change in its perceived loudness and quality. They described changes in their reactions not just to the tinnitus itself but to other aspects of their lives. They found themselves more relaxed, less irritable, and were experienced by their families as being much easier to live with. One in particular felt that her marriage had been greatly improved as a consequence of the improvement in her general mental state.

The trial was carried out in three steps, each step consisting of assessment of tinnitus by audiometric matching before and after a session of hypnosis, and a session with myself in which one of three versions of the approach to hypnotic management of tinnitus was applied. Each such step consisted of two sessions, at the first of which the treatment method was introduced and the patient trained in what he or she would have to practise over the following weeks, and at the second, this training was reinforced. Each step was followed by a gap of approximately three weeks before moving on to the next step. Each treatment method was given to every patient but in different orders. The ENT Department had no knowledge of what went on in the hypnosis sessions, and I (the hypnotherapist) had no information concerning the ratings carried out on the tinnitus.

The treatment methods were as follows:

1   The induction of the hypnotic trance, suggestions of relaxation of body and mind, suggestions of well-being. The patient was to spend 10 to 20 minutes twice a day in the trance state, using a self-hypnosis routine that was taught at the first session and reinforced at each subsequent meeting.

2   Whilst in the hypnotic trance, suggestions were made of a reduction in the loudness of the tinnitus, using an image identified by the patient as appropriate: for example, one patient described his tinnitus as sounding like gas escaping under high pressure from a gas cylinder, and he therefore was to visualise such a cylinder with a valve at the top which he would turn slowly so as to reduce the escape of gas, bit by bit, and therefore reduce the noise.

3   Whilst in the hypnotic trance, suggestions were made of a cessation of the noise, again using imagery that was acceptable to each patient. For example, an electrical engineer

found it good to visualise a bank of electrical switches which he would operate, in imagination, until he found one that reduced the tinnitus; a retired receptionist was happier with the image of an old-fashioned switch board from which she would remove the plugs, one at a time until the tinnitus had stopped.

As indicated at the beginning of this report, not one of the patients seemed to experience a cessation of the noise, and only one experienced a significant reduction in loudness. As far as one can conclude from a relatively small series, and the limitations of a single practitioner, it seems that a significant attack on tinnitus by suggestion under hypnosis does not seem to be of much use, if any at all. Nevertheless, the emotional stress on the patient set up by tinnitus and the effects on the family of the common consequences of tinnitus such as irritability, depression etc., do seem to be to some extent and in some people modifiable by the use of hypnosis.

There is a question that puzzles me about this. Why is it that it is possible to establish under hypnosis total anaesthesia in a 'good hypnotic subject' so that surgery can be carried out without any pain being experienced by the patient, and yet the experience of tinnitus is not blocked by closely similar techniques? It seems that it is possible to 'switch off' the transmission of pain signals from the skin, joints, etc., but not the tinnitus signals. I believe this raises a question as to whether the experience of tinnitus is mediated by nerve transmission from the periphery inwards, or whether the process that results from the experience occurs only centrally, i.e. in the brain itself. Naturally, I would not suggest that the process involved is the same in all cases, and it is well established that some forms of tinnitus are indeed peripherally located.

Some people are able to 'come to terms' with their tinnitus: they 'learn to live with it'. Of the fourteen people who were included in this study, five were helped, by their own accounts, to reach such an adjustment when they had been unable to do so unaided previously. Hypnosis does seem to have a part to play in lessening the distress and disturbance provoked by tinnitus, and it may be that further study could enable us to apply hypnosis more effectively or to identify those people who could be enabled to block out awareness of the noises by the use of this technique.

From the writer's experience in this trial and in other patients, it seems important that anyone undertaking this treatment for tinnitus and expecting the noises to suddenly cease, may very well fail to gain the benefits they *could* have in terms of relaxation, peace of mind, reduction of irritability and so on that can be achieved by the use of hypnosis.

*Hellmut Karle*

## YOGA

This can certainly enhance one's sense of physical well-being and relax both the body and the mind, and as such can be most helpful to many people suffering from tinnitus in which the need for relaxation plays an important part, but of course it must in no way be regarded as a replacement for ordinary medical care.

Hatha Yoga is the type most widely practised in the Western World and although it can be performed on your own it is best to start under a fully trained teacher. Also, since many readers may well not be in the first bloom of youth, it is advisable to ask your doctor before taking it up; and naturally anyone with physical disabilities or other symptoms should certainly leave it out of their reckoning altogether and explore some less demanding avenue of help.

*Letter:* These noises would have driven me crazy years ago if it had not been for another godsend, the mantra Om Namah Shivaya which I was given to use. So I'd like an opportunity to pass it on to others who would be interested.

Using mantra is of course an ancient form of self-help, a mental yoga with which instead of getting caught up in other sounds, circling thoughts and emotions, you let your attention rest with the special mantra sounds, repeating them over and over again to yourself. You can use it at any time, any place, even sitting on a bus, or as a form of meditation.

And here may I say how delighted I have been to read that other sufferers have found meditation a help too. It's a really powerful technique for reaching that centre of peace and contentment which exists deep inside each one of us – like the still centre within a hurricane.

# VIII

# Living with Tinnitus

## LEARN TO LIVE WITH IT

It is unfortunate that sufferers from tinnitus can all too often find themselves in a hopeless position when seeking advice from their doctor. Far too many G.P.s are inclined to take a very negative attitude to tinnitus, informing the patient 'There is nothing that can be done – you have just got to learn to live with it'. In no way is this an indication of ignorance on their part but more a lack of interest since there is no known cure for the condition. This is an attitude that the British Tinnitus Association is trying very hard to alter.

Such an approach may perhaps be forgiven when one realises that the investigation and therapy of tinnitus takes far more time than the average G.P. could possibly hope to devote to it. However, in view of the recent advances in diagnostic techniques and most especially in tinnitus masking, it is a great pity that this attitude should exist, for the referral of a patient to the proper quarter could in so many cases help someone to lead a fuller and happier life.

*Letter:* I have suffered from tinnitus since I was thirteen. I am now forty. I have seen numerous G.P.'s and paid heavily for private consultations with ENT specialists, only to receive the same comments as many readers, namely I must 'learn to live with it'. As the years go by it becomes increasingly harder to 'live with' and my main reason for writing is to ask if there is a specialist anywhere in the country who fully understands the problems of sufferers, who is prepared to take a real interest, and who would carry out a thorough examination for me?

*Reply:* We receive a number of letters from readers who say that their ENT specialists 'brush them off' and do not explain the facts to them. In reply to one such letter our Medical Adviser said:

'ENT surgeons are generally very overworked and see far too many patients, so that they don't have enough time to give to each one. This does not mean necessarily that they do not care; it is simply a symptom of the long-term chronic under-financing of the National Health Service. If you have read all the BTA literature it is possible that you might know more about treatment of your complaint than your local consultant, as a lot of the information is really quite recent and he may not have had the opportunity to learn about it. Please take this into consideration when you see him. It is unlikely that the newer forms of treatment for tinnitus will be available everywhere at once, as they take a lot of time and money to implement, which brings us back to the financial problems that bedevil the Health Service.'

*Letter:* I am relieved to know that something is being done about tinnitus, however slight. Quite clearly, nothing much is known about this, which is illustrated by the lack of success with my GP and two specialists: my doctor said 'You'll have to learn to live with it' the first specialist's closing remark was 'Don't worry, you'll be alright' and the second specialist agreed that if I had noises in my ears that he wouldn't argue with that!

My problem is partly uncertainty. I know I have noises but is this treatable in any way? I was hoping to read about other people's symptoms and perhaps successful treatments, but this was obviously expecting too much.

*Reply:* It is not really helpful just to compare other people's symptoms and find out who got help from what. There are so many different conditions under the one umbrella of tinnitus that it is not likely that one person's 'successful' treatment would help you. If medicine proceeded along these lines, people would spend their whole lives ingesting vast quantities of useless and sometimes harmful drugs. If possible you should go to a clinic where tinnitus is dealt with in detail.

*Letter:* My tinnitus came on very suddenly. I was so frightened that the doctor prescribed a sedative and later called in a psychiatrist. After much consultation he as good as accused me of imagining all these noises and was about to give me an ECT. My noise was very real. I am now being treated by a specialist. I have not been subjected to loud noises to cause this. What distresses me is that I have to take a 'Mogadon' tablet to be able to sleep.
*Reply:* Tinnitus is not always caused by loud noise, but this is often a feature. I have found about 45% of cases have been exposed to loud noise. Sadly some doctors still do not realise that tinnitus is a very real symptom and consider it to be imagined. Things are changing now and the majority of the medical profession, particularly those who read the journals, will know a great deal about its cause and effect. It is true that some things heard in the head can be a symptom of psychiatric illness, but these are usually very much more organised noises – for instance,

voices speaking recognisable sentences or issuing commands.

*Letter:* Thank you for sending me the literature about tinnitus. I have been suffering with it now for seven years, night and day it never ceases. Now I have read your booklets I do not feel alone. I thought I was going mad and that I had a tumour on the brain (proved negative by a brain scan)... My doctor loses patience when I go to see him because he says there is nothing anybody can do when the inner ear goes. I took your booklets along, but he would not listen and said he had no time to read books, so I said that in one of your booklets it says 'don't be fobbed off by your GP when he says nothing can be done'. I told him about the masker and he said he had never heard of them but still would not look at the booklet, so I am back to square one.

*Reply:* I am very sorry that your general practitioner is not interested in the areas of new treatment for this condition. I am afraid you will need the help of your GP if you are to get any treatment and your only solution in this situation is to consider changing your general practitioner. However, before doing this you must make very sure that there is someone else who is prepared to take you on. If you are an older person you may find this a little difficult. I am sorry I cannot be more helpful, but we get many letters from people in the same dilemma.

## INDUSTRIAL COMPENSATION

It is generally accepted that noise trauma can cause tinnitus, although the condition may not be noticeable until many years after the exposure to such noise. In such an event it naturally makes any claim for compensation extremely difficult.

An approach was made by the British Tinnitus Association in 1983 to the DHSS for tinnitus to be included in the list of disabilities eligible for registration. The DHSS replied that they gave no list of specific disabilities which would qualify for registration as a disabled person. They stated that it was up to the Local Authorities to exercise their own discretion in the matter of registration, guided by the National Assistance Act, plus a medical assessment where appropriate.

A booklet on 'The Code of Practice for Reducing the Exposure of Employed Persons to Noise' is available from Her Majesty's Stationery Office, or booksellers, price £1.50.

*Letter:*   During the last twelve months the noise of tinnitus has become so great and high-pitched that my sleep, appetite and general way of life have changed and at times I just do not want to do anything.

I work as a night telephonist at a Telephone Exchange but feel I cannot continue with this type of work. The specialist at the ENT Department told me nothing can be done. The Post Office doctor said much the same thing and that I would have to live with it.

I applied at my local DHSS office for industrial benefit but was told that tinnitus is not recognised as an industrial disease and was not listed. I have therefore applied for a disability benefit and have completed a claim form. Could you advise me if I am entitled to any benefits at all or if something can be done for people like myself? I feel that the type of job I am doing has caused the increase of tone which is now persistent. (We are of course subjected to loud noises at times such as children screaming or whistling or shouting in the mouthpiece when answering calls). I have asked this question but cannot get a 'yes' or a 'no'. Have I a right to claim if I am deemed unable to continue in my job and discharged on medical grounds?

*Reply:*   Awards have been made for tinnitus as a result of industrial noise exposure, but it is often difficult to prove the tinnitus was due to your work as a telephonist. In most of the cases where awards have been made there is considerable deafness as well, and the plaintiff has worked in say, a drop-forge factory for twenty or thirty years.

Although we all experience loud noises down the telephone from time to time, and telephonists more frequently than others, the actual duration of the loud noise is only a very short proportion of your working day. If this sort of noise level had been continuous for eight hours a day, five days a week for many years, then you would definitely have a case.

The problem is that tinnitus is a very common condition, affecting around 17% of the population, and many of these people will be telephonists or exposed to noise at some time. That does not mean that their jobs were necessarily responsible, and that is why it is so difficult to make awards on this ground alone.

*Letter:*   In Newsletter 13 reference was made to the difficulties being encountered by a night telephonist employed by the Post Office Corporation who suffers from tinnitus. Your correspondent applied to the local office of the DHSS for industrial injury benefit and was quite properly told that tinnitus is not a prescribed industrial disease.

I should perhaps explain that for some fifteen years or so I have been dealing with cases of acoustic trauma (frequently associated with tinnitus) amongst our members employed in the telecommunications area of the Civil Service. Whilst it is true that occupational deafness amongst telecommunications grades generally is not a prescribed industrial disease or condition, it has proved possible in a number of cases to establish that the condition was occupationally induced as a result of an industrial injury.

There is an important distinction between injury by 'accident' and injury by 'process'.

I think it very likely that your correspondent is a member of the Union of Communications Workers in the Post Office and I would strongly urge the telephonist concerned to consult her trade union who may be able to offer the member concerned the sort of industrial injury advice or assistance which we extend to our members. . . . The Civil Service Union has been in the forefront of the efforts being made via the Trade Union Congress to persuade the Industrial Injuries Advisory Committee to include tinnitus in the list of prescribed industrial diseases.

*Letter:*   I worked for 14 years as a Cook Supervisor. I had no office and had to do my bookwork four feet from the sink and sterilizing unit where at times 500 plates, 1000 pieces of cutlery and 300 glasses were washed and sterilized daily. I repeatedly asked my superiors if they could insulate my desk or build an office. It was always put off.

About three years ago I started having trouble with my ears. After several consultations with my doctor, he referred me to an ENT specialist who eventually told me he had done all he could and said that I would have to learn to live with the permanent noise I have and that there was no cure for it. He was sure my job was the cause of it.

I wondered if I ought to be considered for a small pension. If this horrible noise is caused through my noisy work, can I claim anything? If so, how do I go about it?

*Reply:*   It is possible to claim against previous employers for tinnitus if this can be shown to be due to noise to which you were exposed. I should warn you that you must first engage a solicitor to act for you, and this might involve getting legal aid, and also quite possibly appearing in court. There have been some very substantial settlements for tinnitus as a result of noise exposure but I'm afraid that I cannot tell you whether the dishwasher which you sat next to would come into this category. As tinnitus is so common, it is very often the case that somebody who was going to develop tinnitus anyway, does so not necessarily as a direct consequence of the noise to which they have been previously exposed.

*British Tinnitus Association leaflet*

## INDUSTRIAL DEAFNESS & TINNITUS

### Assessment of Damages

The assessment of hearing loss for the purpose of assessing damages should be based on both subjective measures (the effect on the sufferer's daily life) and objective measurements (eg the degree of hearing loss measured by audiometry). Objective measurements should take account of hearing loss at high frequencies where most hearing loss occurs and not only that at lower frequencies, as has been the case in many damages awards. Thus, in *Johnson and Ors v the Ministry of Defence* which concerned the amount of damages to be awarded to five employees of the Royal Naval Dockyards, Devonport, Mr Justice Bristow, sitting in the Queen's Bench Division of the High Court at Exeter on 19.3.82, reinforced Mr Justice Mustill's opinion in *Heslop v Metalock Limited* [see above] that objective measurements of hearing loss based only on measurements at frequencies lower than 4kHz were inappropriate. He also took account of the case of *Smith v British Rail Engineering Ltd* which is accepted as a leading case on the issue. There was no transcript of the *Heslop* judgment available at the time of the hearing, but an expert witness common to both cases (Mr Ellis Douek, Consultant Otologist at Guy's Hospital) was able to assist the judge.

The Ministry of Defence had admitted liability for the deafness and tinnitus of the five men who had been employed at the dockyard for periods ranging from 15 to 34 years; the only issue to be decided was the heads and amounts of damages.

In his judgment, Mr Justice Bristow stated that: 'The concensus of evidence before me was that the significant frequency to consider in any comparative analysis of loss of hearing ability in people in ordinary life is 4kHz. The measured difference in loss at this frequency is the only objective basis on which you can make a comparison. . .'. He thus rejected the use of the Coles-Worgan scale [see *Heslop* casenote above] for assessing auditory handicap: 'All these expert witnesses called before me considered it as an unsatisfactory approach to the problem of evaluating the effect on individual patient's enjoyment of life by reason of hearing loss, though no doubt useful for the widely different purposes for which it was designed. I have therefore disregarded it in assessing damages.'

Objective assessments needed to be supplemented by subjective considerations, however. The judge went on to say that the same amount of hearing loss affects different people differently: for example, a social recluse might not ever 'suffer' at all.

In considering the damages to be awarded to each of the five, the judge considered pain and suffering and loss of the amenities of life to be the relevant heads. As there was no significant risk that any of the five were ever likely to lose their jobs, the judge did not award any compensation for future handicap in the labour market. The five were awarded damages ranging from £6500 to £2500 – a total of £18,000 between them.

## DOES FLYING HAVE AN EFFECT ON TINNITUS?

Many sufferers from tinnitus express considerable anxiety over flying, but an enquiry to their doctor should soon put their mind at rest in the majority of cases, for there are few ear difficulties that totally exclude flying.

There are, however, three recognised rules that may be helpful. Firstly, since most of the difficulties affecting the ears in flying occur when the aircraft begins its descent, be sure that you are awake at this time, since the eustachian tubes do not open as effectively when you are asleep. Secondly, sip a glass of liquid from time to time, and if the ear still does not clear, pinch the nose, close the mouth and blow gently. Thirdly, do try to avoid flying with a bad cold as such an infection swells the eustachian tubes.

It should also be mentioned that pressure changes during flight can have a temporary effect on tinnitus, sometimes making it louder, sometimes diminishing it.

The following very useful set of letters and replies on this subject appeared in one of the B.T.A's Newsletters and is repeated here with their permission:

### . . . IF YOU ARE PLANNING A PLANE TRIP

A number of readers who suffer from tinnitus have enquired about travelling by plane. We are publishing the most common questions below, with replies from the Medical Adviser to 'Hearing' to guide those considering air travel:

*Letter:*   I have tinnitus and a perforated ear. Will air travel affect this?
*Reply:*   There is no problem if you have a perforation of the ear drum. In fact you are better off than someone who has an intact ear drum because the pressure can equalise through the hole in the ear drum, rather than up the eustachian tube in the normal manner. If you have not seen an ear specialist recently, I suggest you make another visit – sometimes these perforations heal of their own accord.

*Letter:*   Will air travel make my tinnitus worse?
*Reply:*   Most patients with chronic tinnitus have a small abnormality in the inner ear. The small changes of pressure that occur during air travel sometimes have an effect on the middle ear mechanism. This is because air cannot easily travel up the eustachian tubes to equalise the pressure in either side of the ear drum. This sometimes causes a mild conductive deafness and discomfort and because of this, tinnitus may momentarily seem worse. However, once the ears have cleared everything should return to normal. There is no real danger of the inner ear being damaged by the small pressure changes encountered in modern air travel.

*Letter:*   I have an opportunity to go to the U.S.A. but have never flown and am very afraid that flying may affect my tinnitus. Can you advise on any precautions I can take?
*Reply:*   There is no reason why you should not fly. There is no evidence that flying has any effect on your kind of tinnitus. In modern aeroplanes there is very little change of pressure but it is a good idea to clear the ears on descent by gently blowing down the nose with the nostrils closed between finger and thumb.

*Letter:*   My wife suffers from tinnitus. She worked for a number of years as an air stewardess and suffered from blockage in her ears during descents. The tinnitus came about following a particularly bad experience when she flew with a head cold. Various specialists have tended to take the view that the tinnitus has little or nothing to do with her flying activities. Have similar instances come to light?

*Reply:* It is possible that tinnitus relates to some experience when flying, although at this late stage an exact knowledge of the cause of the tinnitus is unlikely to be of any help in finding a solution to it. There is an increasing awareness that pressure changes can bring about, on rare occasions, a rupture of the delicate membranes in the inner ear and a subsequent leak of fluid from the inner ear. Most of these leaks undoubtedly seal themselves again but leave some slight damage behind which may result in nerve deafness or lead to tinnitus.

# IX

# Self-Help

The emotional effect of the onset of tinnitus varies considerably according to the personality of the sufferer. Many people fear they are going mad, especially since others are unable to hear the noise. Others feel they have developed a brain tumour, or even worse.

Overwrought by the intensity and claustrophobic nature of this constant noise in the head, far too many may attempt to take their own lives. It is in these early stages that a sympathetic G.P. can give considerable support and guidance.

It is possible to help oneself in at least relieving some of the misery of tinnitus, but this demands a certain amount of determination.

It is only right and natural that anyone smitten with a handicap such as this should try to learn as much about it as possible and seek out every possibility of help.

As things stand at the present time, with orthodox medicine only able to help if there is some obvious physical cause for a person's tinnitus, the only other course left for the sufferer is to try a masker; yet this device is only of help in a certain proportion of cases, and even then although it may at least alleviate the condition, it will certainly not cure it.


## SOME SIMPLE SUGGESTIONS

(a)   Remember that tinnitus itself will not cause you to go completely deaf, nor will it cause your death, or cause you to lose your reason. It is important that such terrifying thoughts as these should be cleared totally from your mind.
(b)   Do not use sedatives except on the actual advice of your doctor.

(c)   Since tinnitus is the more noticeable when trying to go to sleep in quiet surroundings, sometimes a ticking clock will serve as a masker and enable you to get off to sleep.

(d)   Drill yourself to accept the existence of this noise in the head and then try to completely ignore it.

(e)   Try sleeping with a fairly high build-up of pillows, this can cause less congestion in the head and may make the tinnitus less noticeable.

(f)   Do not smoke at all, and avoid such stimulants as excessive amounts of coffee, etc.

(g)   Avoid becoming overtired, making sure you obtain sufficient rest at all times.

(h)   Do your best to avoid any kind of anxiety or stress, for your auditory system is already tense and thus these things can only exacerbate your tinnitus.

## LOSS OF HEARING

Since this so often occurs as an accompaniment to tinnitus it is one of the first difficulties with which one must try to cope. Unfortunately deafness, unlike blindness, as we all know has little or no appeal to the sympathetic feelings of others. Even on the stage is not blindness the tragedy and deafness the comedy? With even slight loss of hearing it is quite a natural reaction for one to strive to appear 'normal' especially with a disability like this which is capable of such concealment. But beware! It will surely not be long before you are caught out. There will come a time when you will either reply to a question in some absurd way, or appear extremely rude by failing to reply at all.

Probably the most honest and positive approach to the difficulty is to wear a hearing aid if this is required, otherwise when in difficulty have the courage to explain that you are 'hard of hearing' or 'somewhat deaf' and so avoid embarrassment.

Any form of deafness can impose a considerable strain on one's partner and family, for here one is in a situation in which the simplest of remarks often has to be repeated, and the radio and television have to be turned up to a pitch often most unpleasant to those with normal hearing.

There are devices available to eradicate each of these irritating conditions, and it is surely only fair to others that you should take advantage of them. Tinnitus causes both short temper and irritability in its victims, and to be additionally aware that one is imposing a considerable strain on one's nearest and dearest certainly does not help.

## DEPRESSION

Depression and tinnitus are notoriously closely linked, and in numerous cases of suicide in which the basic cause was tinnitus, only depression has been mentioned at the inquest. It is felt that this is a pity, for it could otherwise have the effect of drawing more public attention to the really serious effect that tinnitus can have upon an individual.

Those people who are anxious, depressed, or inclined towards introspection are much more likely to be more conscious of even mild tinnitus than someone with an extrovert personality. Depression is the handmaiden of tinnitus and it has been proved over and over again that relief from the accompanying depression can do much to help relieve tinnitus.

*Letter:* I have had tinnitus for two years and feel frightened of it. It has affected my nerves badly. Sometimes I have to weep to alleviate some of the stress. I have an emotional nature and am inclined to worry a lot. Can you tell me if I am causing things to be worse and if I am not handling myself in the correct way? The doctors seem unconcerned about the noises. I take Activan and Inderal for my nerves.
*Reply:* It sounds as if you are suffering from depression in addition to tinnitus and this is an extremely common combination. It is often difficult to say whether the depression is closely related to tinnitus or whether it is due to other factors. Both tinnitus and depression are common conditions in middle life and may exist separately or together. Depression can sometimes be helped by specific anti-depressive drugs ... I think it is quite likely that the depression you are suffering from is more severe than the tinnitus. ...

Research into the psychological aspects of tinnitus has been in progress for several years at the Royal National Throat, Nose & Ear Hospital in London, and I am extremely grateful to Richard Hallam PhD. the Principal Clinical Psychologist there for his permission to reprint the following report which originally appeared in the B.T.A. Newsletter:

## TINNITUS TOLERANCE – THE PSYCHOLOGICAL ASPECTS

Report of Tinnitus Research at the Audiology
Centre of the Royal National Throat, Nose & Ear
Hospital, London

by

### RICHARD HALLAM PhD

Research into the psychological aspects of tinnitus began in 1981 when Ronald Hinchcliffe, Professor of Audiological Medicine at the Institute of Laryngology and Otology invited Professor Rachman of the Institute of Psychiatry to collaborate on a short project. This research, conducted by Richard Hallam, helped to identify the psychological facets of tinnitus annoyance, apart from the loudness and quality of the noises themselves. It appeared that tolerance of noises was the general rule, and although noises are distressing for virtually all sufferers to begin with, after a period of time they become less annoying and distressing.

A theoretical model of tinnitus tolerance was proposed (Hallam, Rachman & Hinchcliffe 1984). This emphasised the distinction between the noises being *present* and being *heard*. Although tinnitus seems to force itself on our attention, a person is not always aware of it. We believe that this ability to ignore the noises develops naturally in most sufferers but can be helped along by psychological techniques. This may involve helping the person to think differently about the tinnitus or the way he or she copes with it.

The second stage of our research was supported by the

Medical Research Council for three years and is nearing
completion. An additional worker, Simon Jakes, joined the
team, and at the same time an N.H.S. psychological
counselling service was initiated through the appointment of
Lawrence McKenna, a clinical psychologist, to the hospital
staff. The new research had two main aims, the first being to
extend the psychological model by investigating the nature of
annoyance and the factors causing it. The second aim was to
test out different treatment techniques designed to help
tinnitus sufferers come to terms with their problem and cope
with it better.

Investigations into what makes tinnitus annoying have
examined the *loudness* of tinnitus as an obvious place to start.
We have also considered loudness and refined ways of
measuring it objectively by the established method of
loudness matching, and subjectively with various self-
answered scales. However, it is striking that not all sufferers
complain about tinnitus for the same reasons and loudness
may be more relevant in some cases than others. For some,
sleep is difficult, while others are bothered only during the
day and sleep normally. Some find that tinnitus interferes
with their ability to hear what's being said at parties or
meetings, while others are merely worried because they think
the noises are going to affect their physical or mental health.

Our work so far indicates that there are three main types of
difficulty arising out of tinnitus. These are the *emotional
effects* especially irritability, helplessness and depression,
which result mainly from the way the tinnitus is thought
about by the sufferer, for example as a problem that will never
go away and from which there is little relief.

The emotion of anxiety arises especially from worries that
there is something seriously wrong with the body, or that the
noises will cause a nervous breakdown.

The second type of difficulty is more like a handicap than a
form of emotional distress. It is the effect of tinnitus on one's
ability to listen to and understand, meaningful sounds (over
and above any hearing loss that may be present) and shows
itself in difficulty of localising sounds, distortion of voices,
hearing what's being said against a background noise and
concentrating on mental activities.

The third type of difficulty is getting to sleep and staying asleep.

Our researchers have told us that these three main types of difficulty can be quite independent, so that a person may have one but not the others. How does the loudness of tinnitus fit into this pattern?

We suspect that the loudness of tinnitus is most important in the ability to listen to and focus in on the important events around us including our own thoughts. Loudness may not be so important in causing the emotional effects of tinnitus. It certainly seems true that people can be upset by very quiet noises and ignore very loud ones (or even enjoy them). This is undoubtedly true of external sounds. The emotional effects of tinnitus seem to be more closely related to the attitudes we hold about tinnitus and the meaning we give to it.

The ideas we have developed about tinnitus have been borne out in our work on counselling and therapy. It seems that many of the people we see learn to tolerate tinnitus better even if the loudness and quality of the noises have not changed.

Our first experiment into treatment proved worthless. This was based on the idea that tolerance of the noises could be developed by encouraging the sufferer to listen to external sounds, matched to the pitch of the tinnitus noise. We expected that the ability to switch off attention (interest) in these sounds would transfer to the noises, but this did not happen.

Our second set of experiments was based on the belief that relaxing while listening to the noises, and also switching attention from the noises, would aid tolerance. Relaxation was taught systematically and our patients were encouraged to 'accept' the noises and to use relaxation as a means of coping with them, especially if they had difficulty sleeping.

Our results here were much more promising and we will shortly publish results of the work. Relaxation training, including the biofeedback form of training has been tried elsewhere and found to be beneficial. Our study on 24 chronic tinnitus sufferers has reinforced this view but has also provided more detailed information about the changes it produced. Distraction techniques apparently added nothing of value to relaxation alone.

Patients were seen once a week for five weeks. From two weeks before treatment began until one month after treatment finished they kept daily records of (i) how loud and (ii) how annoying their tinnitus was. We found that although there was a slight decrease in how loud the patients rated their tinnitus, the decrease in annoyance was much greater. The decrease did not begin until relaxation training was started and then it occurred quite rapidly.

Other measures, including ratings of sleep, also changed, especially the worrying thoughts patients expressed about the noises. We have only slight evidence that tinnitus is perceived as less loud in the long run but we believe that as distress is reduced, it becomes possible to pay less attention to the noises so that even the effects on listening and mental concentration are eventually reduced. About half of our patients said that the noises were less annoying but considering that most of them had tried alternative treatments without success, we feel we have made a very good beginning.

Naturally enough, we are already thinking about the next stage. Simon Jakes has obtained a two-year grant from the N.H.S. to compare the effects of maskers with psychological techniques. We would like to develop our ideas on the ways that attitudes to tinnitus, and methods of coping with it, can be changed to benefit the sufferer. We have already experimented with group methods, and enlisted the help of an ex-tinnitus sufferer whose comments are very persuasive. Whether we can continue these initiatives is very much in the balance and awaits the outcome of further grant applications.

*Richard Hallam*

## A SURPRISING DISCOVERY

One of the most surprising discoveries I have made in my researches on tinnitus has been that there are people living today who have obviously been suffering from this condition since birth and in consequence believed that this was a normal and natural part of life and that everyone else heard these noises.

I quote from but two letters from such people taken from the correspondence pages of the B.T.A. newsletters:

*Letter:* My earliest memories were of the noise in my head and many childhood nightmares were centred around it, which was and still is a very high pitched 'electrical whine'. I have never thought anything of it until my late 20s and assumed it was what everyone else heard as well! It was then that I learned about tinnitus!

*Letter:* I have always had head noises – a hissing in the right ear and a howling wind in the left – but it may amaze you to know that I was *sixty years of age* before I discovered that it was not normal to have noises in the head, and that other humans did not experience the same thing.

# X

# 'Hums' – Low Frequency Tinnitus or Environmental Noise?

A few years ago it came to the notice of the media that some two thousand people around Britain were experiencing a continuous low-pitched throbbing hum. The phenomenon is nothing new. Throughout history one can find anecdotes of strange humming and buzzing noises heard by various individuals, and for many years people have from time to time written to newspapers with similar complaint, of noises, many feeling that some vibrational energy is being created by something or someone causing audible sound to them. The name 'pseudo-tinnitus' has even been given to the phenomenon, pointing out that normal tinnitus *and* this environmental sound can both be heard at the same time.

When George Martin published a feature on the problem in the *Sunday Mirror* in 1977 nearly a thousand letters from sufferers were received by the paper; a similar number of letters followed on John Clare's article on the same subject in the *News of the World* in 1979.

The Physics Department of Chelsea College then undertook a thorough investigation. The College was put in touch with a number of people suffering the worst effects of these low humming noises, and these people co-operated by taking part in lengthy interviews and fairly exhaustive tests in an effort to uncover the cause of the problem.

During this investigation most of the people involved reported closely similar experiences. When first aware of the hum they assumed it to be from a diesel lorry with the engine idling over, somewhere in the distance, but after a while since the noise persisted they began to comment on it to others, but then discovered that no one else could hear it. With the hum still continuing they naturally became anxious and after a while a number of them were found to be making enquiries through not only their local authorities, but water boards, electricity authorities, gas companies and the like.

Each said that they experienced considerable frustration over the problem, and although they found relatives and friends perfectly sympathetic, with others being so entirely unable to hear the noise which was so real to them, the situation quite naturally caused them considerable frustration and stress.

The Royal National Throat Nose & Ear Hospital then joined in, and following further investigation it was stated that the majority of these 'hum cases' were suffering from what is known as Low Frequency Tinnitus, but the problem of the others still remained unsolved.

Hum-matching tests were undertaken on the lines used at the R.N.I.D. and the investigators were very surprised at the obvious loudness of the hum being heard by the complainants indicative of the misery this constant loud noise must be causing them.

At around the time I began my researches for this book a certain East Anglian village hit the news with reports of numerous complaints of 'humming' and this was followed by a television programme which unfortunately treated the subject in rather too light a vein.

I met several of the complainants and had long talks with them, but although I suffer from tinnitus myself was quite unable to hear the noise of which they complained. The people I spoke to were intelligent, sensitive, down to earth individuals and could in no way be described as 'cranks'. The majority describe the noise as a very deep toned steady throbbing hum which appears to be loudest at night. Each stated that the noise started suddenly, but there was no connection with the times of starting with other sufferers in the same district.

Very few sufferers report the finding of a really hum-free zone. It is heard in other places besides the home, including when on holiday, and some told me that when going on holiday they are free of sound for some hours on arrival at their destination, but it then returns and they put this down to the 'desensitising' of their hearing due to the noise of the car, train or plane in which they have been travelling. This is rather similar to the temporary relief obtained by some tinnitus sufferers after the use of a masker.

Quite a number of these people complain of a feeling of vibration through the floors, or furniture of the room, and during tests of low-frequency audiometry some sufferers stated that they felt the same kind of vibration, although nothing was sensed by the testers.

Most sufferers from humming have their own ideas of the cause, and accusations are usually aimed at factories, gas and electricity authorities, defence establishments connected with radar, building sites, public utilities and so on.

Although many 'hum' sufferers approach their doctors for help in sleeplessness and depression, it appears that few mention the humming. Consequently tranquillisers and sedatives are prescribed whilst the true cause is overlooked. Similarly, very few will mention tinnitus and then usually only to deny having it.

Since so many of these people talk of suicide and quite a number attempt it, the condition is obviously serious and it is a great pity that more cannot be done for them.

In the absence of any official explanation, neighbours are often the subject of blame, whilst others with imagination refer to extra-terrestial and supernatural causes, these references unfortunately being lapped up by the popular press with a style of reporting that can be so damaging to any serious research and totally unfair to the majority of sufferers who are perfectly sincere in their complaints.

It is well known that many authorities are put to considerable inconvenience and expense in an effort to discover the source of sounds complained of, but in most cases such efforts must be quite fruitless from the start since they would have no specialised equipment or expertise needed for a study of the subject. A certain amount of research has admittedly been done, but the whole matter needs to be studied in considerable depth using the most modern equipment available.

# XI

# The British Tinnitus
# Association

At the inaugural meeting of the British Tinnitus Association held on July 9th 1979 in a committee room at the House of Commons attended by over 200 people, including many important figures in the world of hearing, the Rt Hon Jack Ashley, CH MP welcomed the initiative of the Royal National Institute for the Deaf in setting up this Association, and added that it was one of the most crowded meetings he had seen in this committee room.

In an impassioned speech Jack Ashley said:

'It has been estimated that some two million people suffer from tinnitus. But of course when I put a parliamentary question down about this, the answer was that the Government doesn't know! And this is a fact, that no one knows how many people suffer from tinnitus – which is a staggering indictment of the neglect that this very under-rated malady has been accorded in the past. . . . I think that the measure of distress is shown in the letters and from the people I meet. It is the roaring and the shrieking and the whistling that people have, and doctors tell them they have got to learn to live with it. This is always the answer that people seem to get and I think it is very sad indeed that some people are driven to distraction, and some people write about committing suicide, and still they are told to learn to live with it, which I think is absolutely appalling – and one of the reasons why my wife and I are so determined to see that something is done about it. . . .'

The British Tinnitus Association functions under the auspices of the Royal National Institute for the Deaf and its aim is to focus attention upon the distressing condition of tinnitus. Up until April 1984 it issued a well produced and most interesting quarterly newsletter which contained details of all the latest researches, with correspondence columns (from which so many letters have been quoted in this work) and contained a wide variety of information on tinnitus, together with reports of the many Local Self-Help Groups that have been set up throughout the country.

As from June 1984 the B.T.A's Newsletter has appeared in a special section of the new quarterly Journal of the R.N.I.D. quarterly *Soundbarrier* which goes out to some 65,000 readers. There have been advantages in this new arrangement as this journal carries many articles and much information of additional interest to tinnitus sufferers.

All details of the Association can be obtained from:
The Co-ordinator,
British Tinnitus Association,
105 Gower Street,
London WC1E 6AH
(Tel 01 -387 8033)

# Local Groups and Contacts

AS AT FEBRUARY 1988

*Aberdeen*
Mrs M Hay
Centre for the Deaf
Smithfield Road
AB2 2NR (494566)

*Aberystwyth*
Mrs V Scurlock
5 Trefaenor
Comins-Coch, Aberyswyth
Dyfed SY23 3UB (0970 4796)

*Ashford Middx*
Mrs K Coxon
76 Stanley Road
Ashford Middx
(07842 53884)

*Basildon*
Mrs P Davie
14 Dukes Road
Billericay Essex
(Bas 24985)

*Basingstoke*
Mrs K Pooles
Yew Tree Cottage
20 Wooton St Lawrence
Nr Basingstoke
Hants

*Bangor N Ireland*
Miss I Patterson
8 Ambleside Road
Bangor, Co. Down

*Bath*
Miss F Watts
Hearing Therapist
Royal United Hosp (N)
Combe Park
Avon BA1 3NN

*Bedford*
Mr J Harris
104 Exeter Walk
Bedford
BK41 8QF

*Belfast*
Mrs S Callen
Beechbank House
11 Derryvolgie Avenue
Belfast BT9 6FL

*Birmingham*
Mr E Trowsdale
3 Pilkington Avenue
Sutton Coldfield
B72 1LA
(021–355 1496)

*CORNWALL*
*Boscastle*
Mrs M J Saunders
The Old Post House
Boscastle PL35 0AX

Mrs K Beazley
Lynoweth, Little Lane
Hayle
(756018)

*Boston–Lincs*
Mrs A M Padley
46 Quadring Road
Donington
Spalding PE11 4TD

*Bourne End Bucks*
Mr D C Stedman
7 Cressington Place
Bourne End SL8 5SN
(20691)

*Bournemouth*
Mr H Hood
2 Chine Lodge
80 West Cliff Road
Bournemouth, Dorset

*Bradford*
Mrs J Howorth
23 Sellerdale Avenue
Wyke, W Yorks

*Bridlington*
Miss B J Saunderson
10 Easton Road
Bridlington
N Humberside
(670151)

*Brierley Hill Dudley*
Refer to HQ

*Brighton*
Mr J W Hillson-Mitchell
Stanley House
116 High Street
Rottingdean, Sussex BN2 7HF
(Brighton 309244)

*Bristol*
Mrs B Drake
15 Burfoot Road
Stockwood, Avon
(0272 838128)

*Bury St Edmunds*
Mr P Haymes
10 Barons Road
Bury St Edmunds
Suffolk (705428)

*Cambridge*
Mr V Merryweather
55 Corrie Road
Cambridge CB1 3QQ
(0223 244957)

*Canterbury*
Mrs J Ford
114 New Dover Road
Canterbury CT14 3EJ
(64020)

*Cardiff*
Refer to HQ

*Chelmsford*
Mrs M Lawrence
55 Derwent Way, White Court
Braintree Essex
(0376 29381)

*Chesterfield*
Miss C Wootton
Hearing Therapist
Chesterfield Royal Hosp
Calow S44 5BL
(77271 Ex 2129 pm)

*Cheltenham*
Mr D Bennett
19 The Avenue
Charlton Kings
Cheltenham GL53 9BL

*Cromer/Sheringham*
Mr L Sheppard
'Wingfield'
Sustead Road
Lower Gresham
Norfolk NR11 8RE
(026377 285)

*Crosby–Liverpool*
Miss S Knight
51 Kingsway
Waterloo L22 4RG
(051–928 3269)

*Darlington*
Mr C Marsh
105 Hammond Drive
Darlington
Co Durham

*Dorchester*
Mrs E Crook
7 All Saints Road
Dorchester, Dorset

*Dundee*
Mrs G W Booth
Audiology Dept
Ninewells Hospital
Ninewells DD1 9SY
(0382 60111 Ex 2824)

*Dunfermline*
Mrs J Short
9 Hawthorn Bank
Carnoch
KY12 9JS

*Durham*
Mr H V Gibson
50 Oswald Court
Durham City DH1 3DJ

*Eastbourne*
Mrs M A Constable
6 Short Brow Close
Lower Willingdon
E Sussex BN22 0QX

*East Lancs*
Mr C H W Banger
36 Rainhall Crescent
Barnoldswick
Lancs BB8 6BS
(0282 816775)

*E Molesey Surrey*
Mrs M Offor
32 Spring Gardens
E Molesey KT8 OJA
(01–941 6162)

*Edinburgh*
Miss I Shand
108 Crewe Road West
Edinburgh EH5 2PE
(031–552 1310)

*Enfield*
Refer to HQ

*Epsom*
Mrs M Wilson
207 Hook Road
Epsom, Surrey
(24370)

*Exeter*
Mr H Unsworth
29 Belgrave Road
Newton Abbot
Devon

*Exmouth Devon*
Mr B Moseley
24A Morton Cres
Exmouth EX8 1BG

*Fort William*
Mr A Johnstone
Lanark Place
Fort William
Inverness-shire

*Fylde Coast Lancs*
Miss M Leach
Tregarth
55 Croston Road
Garstang, Preston

*Gloucester*
Mrs J Clarke
66 Laynes Road
Hucclecote
Gloucester GL3 3PY

*Gwynedd*
Mrs J A Wiliamson
Cartref
5 Cae Braenar
Holyhead LL65 2PN

*Havering Essex*
Mr D Clark
6 Nelms Close
Hornchurch, Essex
(04024 41708)

*Hemel Hempstead*
Mrs E Peel
48 High Street
Hemel Hempstead HP1 3AF

*Henley-on-Thames, Berks*
Mr C Holliday
Long Meadow
The Coombe, Streatley

*Hereford*
Mr F J Walsh
54 Prospect Walk
Hereford HR1 1PA

*Hinckley–Leics*
c/o Mr F Lowe
Leicester Group

*Hull*
Mr W Howard
109 Southella Way
Kirkella, Hull
HU10 7LZ

*Inverness*
Mrs F Atkins
17 Manse Road
Nairn, IV12 4RW

*Isle of Wight*
Mrs Lowden
Pixies Place, Hamstead Road
Cranmore, Yarmouth, I.O.W.
(760 862)

*Kenton Devon*
Mr J A Chettle
Peacock Cottage
East Town, Kenton
EX6 8NH

*Kettering*
Mr H C Hitchings
317 Stamford Road
Kettering, Northants
(521962)

*Leeds*
Mrs H Brien
26 Ashfield Close
Crossgates
Leeds, LS15 8JT

*Leicester*
Mr F Lowe
Leicester & County Mission for
the Deaf
135 Welford Road
Leicester LE2 6BE

*Lincoln*
Mrs K Hand
Woodleigh
97 Wragby Road
Lincoln LN2 4PG
(0522 25766)

*Liverpool*
Mrs J Pritchard
PMT Audiology Dept
The Royal Liverpool Hospital
Prescott Street
Liverpool L7 8XP
(051–7090141 Ex. 2162)

*LONDON*
*NW London*
Mr J Shapiro
100 Brim Hill
London N2 0EY
(01–444 9657)

*West London*
Mr V Wooster
86 Cedar Grove
Ealing, London W5 4AR
(01–567 0827)

*SE1 London*
Miss L Gaunt
Hearing Therapist
St Thomas' Hospital
London SE1
(01-928 9292)

*Westminster SW1*
Mrs V Barnett
7 Upper Tooting Park Mansions
Marius Road
London SW17 7QR
(01–673 6439)

*Woolwich SE18*
Mr M O'Toole
15 Wrottesley Road
London SE18
(01–317 8934)

*Maidstone*
Mr L Johnson
71 Reculver Walk
Maidstone
ME15 8SZ
(0622 53399)

*Manchester*
Mr S Etherington
20 Norfolk Close
Cadishead
Manchester M30 5HN

*Mansfield*
Mr B Fox
38 Booth Crescent
Bull Farm Estate
Mansfield NG19 7LG
(0623 651038)

*Middlesbrough*
Mrs R E Flannigan
22 Egerton Street
Middlesbrough
TS1 3LU

*Milton Keynes*
Mr & Mrs Welham
15 St Catherines Avenue
Bletchley
Bucks

*Nottingham*
Mrs C Greaves
17 Rosedale Road
Bakersfield
NG3 7GQ
(865431 or 412878)

*Oxford*
Mr P Steedman
46 Mortimer Drive
Old Marston, Oxford

*Peterborough–Cambs*
Mr A Cruickshank
14 Carleton Crescent
Walton, PE4 6HF

*Plymouth*
Mrs P Ridgeway
8 Almeria Court
Plymouth PL7 3TX

*Portsmouth*
Mr N Clarke
72 Carlton Road
Porchester
Fareham PO16 8JH

*Ripley–Derbys*
Mrs G Wray
5 Laurel Avenue, Ripley
DE5 3PE

*Rochdale*
Mrs M Burr
5 Oak Street Ealees
Littleborough OL15 0HH
(78926)

*Rugby*
Mr R Davis
105 Bilton Road
Rugby
CV22 7AS

*Runcorn*
Mr R Hampson
2 Stone Barn Lane
Palacefields, WA7 2QE

*St Albans*
Mrs J Dyer
154 Hazelwood Drive
St Albans

*Salisbury*
Mrs M Coles
12 Vicarage Gardens
Salisbury SP4 9RW
(0980 70718)

*Scalby N Yorks*
Mr R Welburn
4 South Street, Scalby

*S E Northumberland*
(Choppington)
Mr & Mrs R Lillico
10 Simonside Avenue
Stakeford
(Ashington 813726)

*Sevenoaks*
Mrs K M Lee
30 Dartford Road
Sevenoaks, Kent
DN13 3TQ

*Sheffield*
Miss M Scarr
34 Chesterwood Drive
Sheffield S10 5DU

*Sidmouth*
Mrs J Webb
46 Harcombe Lane East
Sidford, Sidmouth
Devon EX19 9RP

*Southampton*
Miss S Graham
24 Launcelyn Close
North Baddesley
Southampton SO52 9NP

*Stevenage*
Mr J C Wilkinson
16 Rockingham Way
Stevenage SG1 1SG

*Stoke-on-Trent*
Mr R F Tizley
Ellis Memorial Centre
Wellesley Street
Shelton, Staffs
(29161)

*Sunderland*
Mr J G Shepherd
20 Corbett Street
Seaham SR7 0AW

*Swansea*
Mrs J Michael
2 Mayals Avenue
Mayals
Swansea, Glamorgan

*Swindon*
Mr C Humber
23 Tavistock Road
Park North, Swindon

*Taunton*
Mr P Besley
Area Soc Ser Officer
Huntscourt
17 Corporation Street
Taunton TA1 4DH

*Tunbridge Wells*
Mr D Watts
177 Forest Road
Tunbridge Wells
Kent TN2 5JA
(0892 27513)

*Wakefield*
Mr R Mitchell
7 Crimble Clough
Slaithwaite
Huddersfield HD7 5DA

*Weston-Super-Mare*
Mrs N Attwell
Hearing Therapist
Weston Gen Hospital
The Boulevard
Weston-super-Mare
Somerset
(0934 25211 Ex 55)

*Wigan*
Mrs S Cowburn
Bank House, Thorn Hill
Boarshead, Wigan WN1 2RS

*Wirral*
Mr W E Griffiths
4 Meadway
Lower Village, Heswall
Merseyside L60 8PH

*Wolverhampton*
Mrs M Crooks
58 Lawnside Green
Bilston, W Midlands
Bilston 46597

*Yeovil*
Mrs J Harris
13 St Margaret's Road
Tintinhull
Somerset BA22 8PL

*York*
Refer to HQ

*Contacts:*

Northampton
Contact Kettering

Reading
Contact Swindon

South Shields
Contact S E Northumberland

Weymouth
Contact Dorchester

Worcester
Contact Hereford

*Overseas Local Groups &*
*Contacts*

*Australia*
Australia Tinnitus Assoc Ltd
288 Unwins Bridge Road
Sydenham
New South Wales 2044

*Canada*
*Toronto*
Mrs E Eayrs
Toronto Tinnitus Group
23 Ellis Park Road
Toronto, Ontario
M6S 2V4

Mr N McDonald
1777 Marquis Avenue
Gloucester K1J 8LS
Canada

*Vancouver*
Mr L Leader
4384 W 12th Ave
Vancouver, B.C.
V6R 2R1

Victoria Tinnitus Assoc
St Ann's Academy
302–835 Humbolt Street
Victoria, B.C. V8V 2M4

*Eire*
*Cork City*
Mr J P Smythe
'Ashford'
Donovans Road
Cork

*Dublin*
Mr Pearse Ward
111 Ventry Park
Cabra West
Dublin 7.

*New Zealand*
*Christchurch*
Mr B White
61 Sevenoaks Drive
Christchurch 5.

*Auckland*
Mrs J Saunders
31 William Souter St
Auckland

*USA*
American Tinnitus Association
PO Box 5
Portland
Oregon 97207
(503 248 9985)

# Bibliography

A number of the following references have been of invaluable assistance in the preparation of this book.

## TINNITUS

Selected post 1979 references, arranged chronologically.

COCHRAN, J.H. & KOSMICKI, P.W. Tinnitus as a presenting symptom in pernicious anaemia. ANNALS OF OTOLOGY, RHINOLOGY AND LARYNGOLOGY, 1979, 88, 297.

DANESHMEND, T.K. Treatment of tinnitus. BRITISH MEDICAL JOURNAL, 1979, 1(6178), 1628, (Letter).

HARRIS, S. et al. Pulsatile tinnitus and therapeutic embolization. ACTAOTOLARYNGOLOGICA, 1979, 88, 220–226.

HAZELL, J.W.P. Tinnitus. BRITISH JOURNAL OF HOSPITAL MEDICINE, 1979, 22, 468–471.

HAZELL, J.W.P. Tinnitus. In BROWN, W.C. Scott-. Scott-Brown's diseases of the ear, nose and throat. 4th ed., edited by John Ballantyne and John Groves. Vol. 2. The ear. London: Butterworth, 1979, pp. 81–91.

HAZELL, J.W.P. Tinnitus research: the current position. HEARING, 1979, 34, 10–15.

LESINSKI, S.G. et al. Why not the eighth nerve? Neurovascular compression – probable cause for pulsatile tinnitus. OTOLARYNGOLOGY AND HEAD AND NECK SURGERY, 1979, 87, 89–94.

LEVEQUE, H. et al. Tympanometry in the evaluation of vascular lesions of the middle ear and tinnitus of vascular origin. LARYNGOSCOPE, 1979, 89, 1197–1218.

LIND, M G. & LUNDQUIST, P.G. Tinnitus caused by bilateral shunts from the occipital arteries to the intracranial veins. A case report. ARCHIVES OF OTORHINOLARYNGOLOGY, 1979, 222, 229–234.

LONGRIDGE, N.S. A tinnitus clinic. JOURNAL OF OTOLARYNGOLOGY, 1979, 8, 390–395.

MELDING, P.S. & GOODEY, R.J. The treatment of tinnitus with oral anticonvulsants. JOURNAL OF LARYNGOLOGY AND OTOLOGY, 1979, 93, 111–122.

PANG, L.Q. et al. A new method of managing subjective tinnitus. HAWAII MEDICAL JOURNAL, 1979, 38, 235–239.

PORTMAN, E. *et al.* Temporary tinnitus suppression in man through electrical stimulation of the cochlea. ACTA OTOLARYNGOLOGICA, 1979, *87*, 294–299.

RAHKO, T, & HAKKINEN, V. Carbamazepine in the treatment of objective myoclonus tinnitus. JOURNAL OF LARYNGOLOGY AND OTOLOGY, 1979, *93*, 123–127.

TINNITUS. LANCET, 1979, *1*,(8126), 1124. (Editorial)

TREATMENT of tinnitus. BRITISH MEDICAL JOURNAL, 1979, *1*,(6176), 1445–1446. (Editorial)

CARBARY, L.J. Tuning out tinnitus. JOURNAL OF NURSING CARE, 1980, *13*, 8–11.

FORMBY, C. & GJERDINGEN, D.B. Pure-tone masking of tinnitus. AUDIOLOGY, 1980, *19*, 519–535.

GOODWIN, P.E. & JOHNSON, R.M. The loudness of tinnitus. ACTA-OTOLARYNGOLOGICA, 1980. *90*, 353–359.

GOODWIN, P.E. & JOHNSON, R.M. A comparison of reaction times to tinnitus and nontinnitus frequencies, EAR AND HEARING, 1980, *1*, 148–155.

HAZELL, J.W.P. Drug treatment in tinnitus: the present position in Britain. HEARING AID JOURNAL, 1980, *33*(12), 9, 58.

HAZELL, J.W.P. Tinnitus research in the U.S.A.: visit to Portland, Oregon, July 13th–28th, 1980. London: RNID, [1980]. 4p.

LOAVENBRUCK, A. Tinnitus masking devices: safe and effective? ASHA, 1980, *22*, 857–861.

MARTIN, F.W. & COLMAN, B.H. Tinnitus: a double-blind crossover controlled trial to evaluate the use of lignocaine. CLINICAL OTOLARYNGOLOGY, 1980, *5*, 3–11.

MEYERHOFF, W.L. & SHREWSBURY, D. Rational approaches to tinnitus. GERIATRICS, 1980, *35*, 90–93.

MILES, S.W. Amitriptyline side effect. NEW ZEALAND MEDICAL JOURNAL, 1980, *92*, 66–67. (Letter.) PENNER, M.J. Two-tone forward masking patterns and tinnitus. JOURNAL OF SPEECH AND HEARING RESEARCH, 1980, *23*, 779–786.

RACY, J. & WARD-RACY, E.A. Tinnitus in imipramine therapy. AMERICAN JOURNAL OF PSYCHIATRY, 1980, *137*, 854–855.

ROESER, R.J. & PRICE, D.R. Clinical experience with tinnitus maskers. EAR AND HEARING, 1980, *1*, 63–68.

ROSE, D.E. Tinnitus maskers: a follow-up. EAR AND HEARING, 1980, *1*, 69–70.

RUDIN, D.O. Glaucoma, 'auditory glaucoma', 'articular glaucoma' and the third eye. MEDICAL HYPOTHESES, 1980, *6*, 427–430.

SASAKI, C.T. *et al.* Differential (14C)2-deoxyglucose uptake after deafferentation of the mammalian auditory pathway: a model for examining tinnitus. BRAIN RESEARCH, 1980, *194*, 511–516.

SCHLEUNING, A.J. *et al.* Evaluation of a tinnitus masking program: a follow-up study of 598 patients. EAR AND HEARING, 1980, *1*, 71–74.

STACEY, J.S. Apparent total control of severe bilateral tinnitus by masking, using hearing aids. BRITISH JOURNAL OF AUDIOLOGY, 1980, *14*, 59–60.

THE treatment of tinnitus, CLINICAL OTOLARYNGOLOGY, 1980, *5*, 1–2. (Editorial).

TONNDORF, J. Acute cochlear disorders: the combination of hearing loss, recruitment, poor speech discrimination, and tinnitus. ANNALS OF OTOLOGY, RHINOLOGY AND LARYNGOLOGY, 1980, *89*, 353–358.

VERNON, J. *et al.* The characteristics and natural history of tinnitus in Meniere's disease. OTOLARYNGOLOGIC CLINICS OF NORTH AMERICA, 1980, *13*, 611–619.

WALFORD, R.E. Acoustical techniques for diagnosing low-frequency tinnitus in noise complainants known as hummers. PROCEEDINGS OF THE INSTITUTE OF ACOUSTICS, 1980, 3.9. 183–186.

WILLIAMS, J.D. Unusual but treatable cause of fluctuating tinnitus. ANNALS OF OTOLOGY, RHINOLOGY AND LARYNGOLOGY, 1980, *89*, 239–240. WILSON, J.P. Model for cochlear echoes and tinnitus based on an observed electrical correlate. HEARING RESEARCH, 1980, *2*, 527–532.

WILSON, J.P. Evidence for a cochlear origin for acoustic re-emissions, threshold fine-structure and tonal tinnitus. HEARING RESEARCH, 1980, *2*, 233–252.

WILSON, J.P. Recording of the Kemp echo and tinnitus from the ear canal without averaging. JOURNAL OF PHYSIOLOGY, 1980, *298*, 8–9.

BORTON, T.E. *et al.* Electromyographic feedback treatment for tinnitus aurium. JOURNAL OF SPEECH AND HEARING DISORDERS, 1981, *46*, 39–45.

BRENNAN, F.J. & SALERNO, T.A. Surgical treatment of symptomatic cervical venous hum. JOURNAL OF THORACIC AND CARDIOVASCULAR SURGERY, 1981, *81*, 135–136.

CHOUARD, C.H. *et al.* Transcutaneous electrotherapy for severe tinnitus. ACTA OTOLARYNGOLOGICA, 1981, *91*, 415–422.

ELFNER, L.F. *et al.* Effects of EMG and thermal feedback training on tinnitus: a case study. BIOFEEDBACK AND SELF REGULATION, 1981, *6*, 517–521.

EPLEY, J.M. Electronic probe for eustachian tube patency and objective tinnitus. OTOLARYNGOLOGY AND HEAD AND NECK SURGERY, 1981, *89*, 854–855.

EVANS, D.L. & GOLDEN, R.N. Protriptyline and tinnitus. JOURNAL OF CLINICAL PSYCHOPHARMACOLOGY, 1981, *1*, 404–406.

GLASS, R.M. Ejaculatory impairment from both phenelzine and imipramine, with tinnitus from phenelzine. JOURNAL OF CLINICAL PSYCHOPHARMACOLOGY, 1981, *1*, 152–154.

GOODHILL, V. Leaking labyrinth lesions, deafness, tinnitus and dizziness. ANNALS OF OTOLOGY, RHINOLOGY and LARYNGOLOGY, 1981, *90*, 99–106.

HARDISON, J.E. *et al.* Self-heard venous hums. JOURNAL OF THE AMERICAN MEDICAL ASSOCIATION, 1981, *245*, 1146–1147.

HAZELL, J.W.P. & WOOD, S. Tinnitus masking, a significant contribution to tinnitus management. BRITISH JOURNAL OF AUDIOLOGY, 1981, *15*, 223–230.

HAZELL, J.W.P. Tinnitus. PRACTITIONER, 1981, *225*, 1577–1585.

HOUSE, J.W. Management of the tinnitus patient. ANNALS OF OTOLOGY, RHINOLOGY AND LARYNGOLOGY, 1981, *90*, 597–601.

INTERNATIONAL TINNITUS SEMINAR, 1st, New York, 1979. JOURNAL OF LARYNGOLOGY AND OTOLOGY, Supplement 4, 1981.

KAY, N.J. Oral chemotherapy in tinnitus. BRITISH JOURNAL OF AUDIOLOGY, 1981, *15*, 123–124.

McCORMICK, M.S. & THOMAS, J.N. Mexiletine in the relief of tinnitus: a report on a sequential double-blind crossover trial. CLINICAL OTOLARYNGOLOGY, 1981, *6*, 255–258.

MADDOX, H.E. & PORTER, T.H. Evaluation of a tinnitus masker. AMERICAN JOURNAL OF OTOLOGY, 1981, *2*, 199–203.

MAN, A., & NAGGAN, L. Characteristics of tinnitus in acoustic trauma. AUDIOLOGY, 1981, *20*, 72–78.

MARKS, N.J. *et al*. The effect of single doses of amylobarbitone sodium and carbamazepine in tinnitus. JOURNAL OF LARYNGOLOGY AND OTOLOGY, 1981, *95*, 941–945.

MARSH, M.N. *et al*. Tinnitus in a patient with beta-thalassaemia intermedia on long-term treatment with deaferrioxamine. POST-GRADUATE MEDICAL JOURNAL, 1981, *57*, 582–584.

PENNER, M.J. *et al*. The temporal course of the masking of tinnitus as a basis for inferring its origin. JOURNAL OF SPEECH AND HEARING RESEARCH, 1981, *24*, 157–261.

SASAKI, C.T. *et al*. Tinnitus: development of a neurophysiologic correlate. LARYNGOSCOPE, 1981, *91*, 2018–1024.

SHAILER, M.J. *et al*. Critical masking bands for sensorineural tinnitus. SCANDINAVIAN AUDIOLOGY, 1981, *10*, 157–162.

SHEA, J.J. *et al*. Medical treatment of tinnitus. ANNALS OF OTOLOGY, RHINOLOGY AND LARYNGOLOGY, 1981, *90*, 601–609.

SHULMAN, A. & SEITZ, M.R. Central tinnitus – diagnosis and treatment. Observations simultaneous binaural auditory brain responses with monaural stimulation in the tinnitus patient. LARYNGOSCOPE, 1981, *91*, 2025–2035.

SPITZER, J.B. Auditory effects of chronic alcoholism DRUG AND ALCOHOL DEPENDENCE, 1981, *8*, 317–335.

TANGE, R.A. & BERNARD, J.L. A cochlear vascular anomaly in a patient with hearing loss and tinnitus. ARCHIVES OF OTORHINOLARY-NGOLOGY, 1981, *233*, 117–125.

TANGE, R.A. & BERNARD, J.L. Tinnitus, a 2000 Hz dip and a suspension vessel in the scala tympani. CLINICAL OTOLARY-NGOLOGY, 1981, *6*, 300. (Abstract.)

THOMAS, J.E. & CODY, D.T. Neurologic perspectives of otosclerosis. MAYO CLINIC PROCEEDINGS, 1981, *56*, 17–21.

TINNITUS: Ciba Foundation symposium, 85, edited by David Evered and Geralyn Lawrenson, London, 1981. London: Pitman, 1981.

TONNDORF, J. Stereociliary dysfunction, a case of sensory hearing loss, recruitment, poor speech discrimination and tinitus. ACTA OTO-LARYNGOLOGICA, 1981, *91*, 469–479.

YANICK, P. Tinnitus: a holistic approach. HEARING INSTRUMENTS, 1981, *32*(7), 12–15, 39.

AHMAD, R. *et al*. Vancomycin: a reappraisal. BRITISH MEDICAL JOURNAL, 1982, *284* (6333), 1953–1954. (Letter).

CATHCART, J.M. Assessment of the value of tocainide hydrochloride in the treatment of tinnitus. PROCEEDINGS OF THE IRISH OTOLARY-NGOLOGICAL SOCIETY, 1982, 60–63.

COLLARD, M.E. *et al*. Conditioned middle ear muscle tinnitus a case report. ANNALS OF OTOLOGY, RHINOLOGY AND LARYNGOLOGY, 1982, *91*, 330–331.

DECKER, T.M. & FRITSCH, J.H. Objective tinnitus in the dog. JOURNAL OF THE AMERICAN VETINARY MEDICAL ASSOCIATION, 1982, *180*, 74.

HARFORD, E.R. Tinnitus maskers. *In* PAPARELLA, M.M. & GOYOCOOLEA, M.V. (eds) Clinical problems in otitis media and innovations in surgical otology. Baltimore: Williams and Wilkins, 1982. 1–8.

ISRAEL, J.M. *et al*. Lidocaine in the treatment of tinnitus aurium: a double blind study. ARCHIVES OF OTOLARYNGOLOGY, 1982, *108*, 471–473.

IURATO, A, & ZITO, F. Tinnitus suppression in man by electrical stimulation with semipermanent electrode. *In* SYMPOSIUM ON ARTIFICIAL AUDITORY STIMULATION, Erlangen, 1982, Cochlear implants in clinical use: edited by W.D. Keidel and P. Finkenzeller. Basel: S. Karger, 1984. (Advances in Audiology, Vol. 2.) pp. 104–107.

KAUER, J.S. *et al*. Tinnitus aurium: fact or fancy. LARYNGOSCOPE, 1982, *92*, 1401–1407.

MARTIN, F.W. Adaptation of drugs in the management of tinnitus. NEWSLETTER (BRITISH TINNITUS ASSOCIATION), 1982, *18*, i–iii.

MEADOR, K.J. *et al*. Self-heard venous bruit due to increased intracranial pressure. LANCET, 1982, *1*(8268), 391. (Letter)

MORGAN, C. McLeod- *et al*. Cognitive restructuring: a technique for the relief of chronic tinnitus. AUSTRALIAN JOURNAL OF CLINICAL AND EXPERIMENTAL HYPNOSIS, 1982, *10*, 27–33.

PILLING, M. A modified gas-liquid chromatographic assay to monitor plasma mexiletine in a tinnitus study. METHODS AND FINDINGS IN EXPERIMENTAL AND CLINICAL PHARMACOLOGY, 1982, 4, 243–247.

REDDELL, R.R. *et al*. Ototoxity in patients receiving cisplatin: importance of dose and method of drug administration. CANCER TREATMENT REPORTS, 1982, *66*, 19–23.

RIEDNER, & YOUNG, Experience with tinnitus therapy. HEARING INSTRUMENTS, 1982, *33*, 28–

SHREWSBURY, D.W. & MEYERHOFF, W.L. Tinnitus: diagnosis and treatment. *In* PAPARELLA, M.M. & GOYCOOLEA, M.V. (eds). Clinical problems in otitis media and innovations in surgicalotology. Baltimore: Williams and Wilkins, 1982. 113–116.

SVIHOVEC, & CARMEN, Relaxation-biofeed back treatment for tinnitus. HEARING INSTRUMENTS, 1982, *33*, 32–

TURNER, J.S. Treatment of hearing loss, ear pain, and tinnitus in older patients. GERIATRICS, 1982, *37*, 107–11, 116, 118.

UNITED STATES. *Committee on Hearing Bioacoustics and Biomechanics. Working Group 89*. Tinnitus: facts, theories and treatments, by Dennis McFadden. Washington: National Academy Press, 1982.

WALFORD, R.E. Hums and hummers: a bibliography of references to low-frequency tinnitus, vascular and dental processes, muscle tremor, the microwave auditory effect and low-frequency sound and hearing. London: Institute of Laryngology, 1982. 43p.

WOOD, S. Maskers and tinnitus patients. NEWSLETTER (BRITISH TINNITUS ASSOCIATION), 1982, *17*, i–iii.

YANICK, New hope for hearing and tinnitus problems: nutrition and biochemistry. HEARING INSTRUMENTS, 1982, *33*, 34–

BRATTBERG, G. An alternative method of treating tinnitus: relaxation hypnotherapy primarily through the home use of a recorded audio cassette. INTERNATIONAL JOURNAL OF CLINICAL AND EXPERIMENTAL HYPNOSIS, 1983, *31*, 90–97.

BUCKWALTER, J.A. *et al*. Pulsatile tinnitus arising from jugular megabulb deformity: a treatment rationale. LARYNGOSCOPE, 1983, *93*, 1534–1539.

CAHANI, M. *et al*. Tinnitus pitch and acoustic trauma. AUDIOLOGY, 1983, *22*, 357–363.

CHANDLER, J.R. Diagnosis and cure of venous hum tinnitus. LARYNGOSCOPE, 1983, *93*, 892–895.

COLES, R. Tinnitus work in the Institute of Hearing Research. NEWSLETTER (BRITISH TINNITUS ASSOCIATION), 1983, *22*, 2–6.

DAWEERT, L.G. & REES, T.S. Treatment of tinnitus with intravenous lidocaine: a double-blind randomized trial. OTOLARYNGOLOGY: HEAD AND NECK SURGERY, 1983, *91*, 550–555.

EHRENBERGER, K. & BRIX, R. Glutamic acid and glutamic acid diethylester in tinnitus treatment. ACTA OTOLARYNGOLOGICA, 1983, *95*, 599–605.

FELDMANN, H. Time patterns and related parameters in masking of tinnitus. ACTA OTOLARYNGOLOGICA, 1983, *95*, 594–598.

GEORGE, B. *et al*. Tinnitus of venous origin: surgical treatment by the ligation of the jugular vein anastomosis. JOURNAL OF NEURO-RADIOLOGY, 1983, *10*, 23–30.

GOLDEN, R.N. *et al*. Doxepin and tinnitus. SOUTHERN MEDICAL JOURNAL, 1983, *76*, 1202–1205.

HAZELL, J.W.P. & WOOD, S. Drug therapy and tinnitus: the U.K. experience. Paper presented at the 2nd International Seminar, New York, June 1983. (In press Journal of Laryngology and Otology.)

HAZELL, J.W.P. *et al.* Electrical stimulation of the cochlea and tinnitus. Paper presented at the 10th Anniversary Conference on Cochlear Implantation, San Francisco, June 1983. (In press.)

HAZELL, J.W.P. The general Household Survey on Tinnitus. NEWSLETTER (BRITISH TINNITUS ASSOCIATION), 1983, *20*, vii–viii.

HAZELL, J.W.P. Spontaneous cochlear acoustic emissions and tinnitus: clinical experience in the tinnitus patient. Paper presented at the 2nd International Seminar, New York, June 1983. (In press Journal of Laryngology and Otology.)

HAZELL, J.W.P., Tinnitus. MEDICINE INTERNATIONAL, 1983, *1*, 1342–1343.

HAZELL, J.W.P. Tinnitus. MODERN MEDICINE, 1983, *28*, 9–10.

HULSHOF, J.H. Drug therapy of tinnitus: the effect of intravenous lignocaine and oral tocainide on tinnitus. CLINICAL OTOLARYNGOLOGY, 1983, *8*, 433. (Abstract.)

JACKSON, P. Tinnitus in the elderly. *In* HINCHCLIFFE, R. Hearing and balance in the elderly. Edinburgh: Churchill Livingstone, 1983, pp. 159–173.

LINDSAY, M. The roaring deafness. NURSING TIMES, 1983, *79*, 61–63.

MAJUMDAR, B. *et al.* An electrocochleographic study of the effects of lignocaine on patients with tinnitus. CLINICAL OTOLARYNGOLOGY, 1983, *8*, 175–180.

MARCHIANDO, A. Tinnitus due to idiopathic stapedial muscle spasm. EAR, NOSE AND THROAT JOURNAL, 1983, *62*, 4–7.

MITCHELL, C. The masking of tinnitus with pure tones. AUDIOLOGY, 1983, *22*, 73–87.

OFFICE OF POPULATION CENSUSES AND SURVEYS. *General Household Survey*. The prevalence of tinnitus, 1981, by E. Goddard and A. Fenton Lewis. London: OPCS, 1983.

PENNER, M.J. Variability in matches to subjective tinnitus. JOURNAL OF SPEECH AND HEARING RESEARCH, 1983, *26*, 263–267.

ROBINSON, W. New treatment for tinnitus. NEW AGE, 1983, *22*, 34–35.

SALVI, R.J. & AHROON, W.A. Tinnitus and neural activity. JOURNAL OF SPEECH AND HEARING RESEARCH, 1983, *26*, 629–632.

SHAPIRO, J. Tinnitus. TALK, 1983, *108*, 24–25.

SLATER, R. *et al.* Tinnitus survey: initial results from the Tinnitus Research Group, Cardiff. NEWSLETTER (BRITISH TINNITUS ASSOCIATION), 1983, *20*, i–v.

SPITZER, J.B. *et al.* Effect of tinnitus masker noise on speech discrimination in quiet and two noise backgrounds. SCANDINAVIAN AUDIOLOGY, 1983, *12*, 197–200.

TERRY, A.M.P. *et al.* Parametric studies of tinnitus masking and residual inhibition. BRITISH JOURNAL OF AUDIOLOGY, 1983, *17*, 245–256. TEWFIK, S. Phonocephalography and pulsatile tinnitus in a surface cerebral angioma: report of a case. JOURNAL OF LARYNGOLOGY AND OTOLOGY, 1983, *97*, 959–962.

TYLER, R.S. & BAKER, L.J. Difficulties experienced by tinnitus sufferers. JOURNAL OF SPEECH AND HEARING DISORDERS, 1983, *48*, 150–154.

TYLER, R.S. & CONRAD-ARMES, D. The determination of tinnitus loudness considering the effects of recruitment. JOURNAL OF SPEECH AND HEARING RESEARCH, 1983, 26, 59–72.

VERNON, J.A. *et al.* A search for possible physiological correlates of subjective tinnitus. *In* Hearing and other senses: presentation in honor of E.G. Wever; edited by Richard R. Fay and George Courevitch. Groton, Connecticut: Amphora Press, 1983, pp. 385–399.

VIRTANEN, H. Objective tubal tinnitus: a report of two cases, JOURNAL OF LARYNGOLOGY AND OTOLOGY, 1983, 97, 857–862.

WALFORD, R.E. A classification of environmental 'hums' and low-frequency tinnitus. JOURNAL OF LOW FREQUENCY NOISE AND VIBRATION, 1983, 2, 60–84.

WOOD, K.A. *et al.* Intractable tinnitus: psychiatric aspects of treatment. PSYCHOSOMATICS, 1983, 24, 559–561, 565.

YOUNG, I.M. & LOWRY, L.D. Incurrence and alterations in contra-lateral tinnitus following monaural exposure to a pure tone. JOURNAL OF THE ACOUSTICAL SOCIETY OF AMERICA, 1983, 73, 2219–2221. (Letter)

BALOH, R.W. Dizziness, hearing loss and tinnitus: the essentials of neurotology. Philadelphia: F.A. Davis, 1984.

BLAYNEY, A.W. *et al.* A sequential double blind crossover trial of tocainide hydrochloride in tinnitus. CLINICAL OTOLARYNGOL-OGY, 1984, 9, 135. (Abstract.)

BURNS, E.M. A comparison of variability among measurements of subjective tinnitus and objective stimuli. AUDIOLOGY, 1984, 23, 426–440.

CAHANI, M. *et al.* Tinnitus asymmetry. AUDIOLOGY, 1984, 23, 127–135.

CHUNG, D.Y. Factors affecting the prevalence of tinnitus. AUDIOL-OGY, 1981, 23, 441–452.

CLARK, J.G. and YANICK, P. (*eds*) Tinnitus and its management: a clinical text for audiologists. Springfield (Ill.): Charles C. Thomas, 1984. CLAUSSEN, C.F. & CLAUSSEN, E. Objective neural-otological investigations in patients with vertigo and tinnitus using ENG and acoustically evoked responses. ARCHIVES OF OTO-RHONO-LARYNGOLOGY, 1984, 239, 101. (Summary.)

COLES, R.R.A. *et al.* Measurement and management of tinnitus. Part. 1. Measurement. JOURNAL OF LARYNGOLOGY AND OTOLOGY, 1984, 98, 1171–1176.

DAWES, J.D.K. What treatment is advised for a 70 year old patient with severe bilateral tinnitus uncontrolled by prochlorperazine or trif-luoperazine? (Any Questions?). BRITISH MEDICAL JOURNAL, 1984, 289(6436), 42.

DUCKERT, L.G. and REES, T.S. Placebo effect in tinnitus management. OTOLARYNGOLOGY HEAD AND NECK SURGERY, 1984, 92, 697–699.

DUCKRO, P.N. *et al* Comprehensive behavioral management of tinnitus: a case illustration. BIOFEEDBACK AND SELF REGULA-TION, 1984, 9, 459–469.

INCE, L.P. *et al.* Learned self-control of tinnitus through a matching-to-sample feedback technique: a clinical investigation. JOURNAL OF BEHAVIORAL MEDICINE, 1984, 7, 358–365. INTERNATIONAL TINNITUS SEMINAR, 2nd, New York, 1983. Proceedings ... JOURNAL OF LARYNGOLOGY AND OTOLOGY, 1984, Supplement 9.

HALLAM, R. *et al.* Psychological aspects of tinnitus. *In* RACHMAN, S. (ed.) Contributions to medical psychology. 3. Oxford: Pergamon Press, 1984. pp. 31–53.

HOUSE, J.W. Tinnitus: evaluation and treatment. AMERICAN JOURNAL OF OTOLOGY, 1984, 5, 472–475.

HULSHOF, J.H. and VERMIJ, P. The effect of intra-venous lidocaine and several different doses oral tocainide HC1 on tinnitus: a dose-finding study. ACTA OTO-LARYNGOLOGICA, 1984, 98, 231–238.

HVIDEGAARD, T. and BRASK, T. Objective venous tinnitus: a case report. JOURNAL OF LARYNGOLOGY AND OTOLOGY, 1984, 98, 189–191.

LAMPRECHT, J. and MORGENSTERN, C. A simple method for the differentiation of tonal tinnitus. ARCHIVES OF OTO-RHINO-LARYNGOLOGY, 1984, 239, 120. (Summary.)

LARSSON, B. *et al.* Tocainide and tinnitus. ORL, 1984, 46, 21–33.

LECHTENBERG, R. and SMULMAN, A. The neurologic implications of tinnitus. ARCHIVES OF NEUROLOGY, 1984, 41, 718–721.

LINDBERG, P. *et al.* Tinnitus: incidence and handicap. SCANDINAVIAN AUDIOLOGY, 1984, 13, 287–291.

LYTTKENS, L. *et al.* Local anaesthetics and tinnitus: proposed peripheral mechanism of action of lidocaine. ORL, 1984, 46, 17–23.

MARKS, N.J. *et al.* A controlled trial of acupuncture in tinnitus. JOURNAL OF LARYNGOLOGY AND OTOLOGY, 1984, 98, 1103–1109.

MAY, J. Tinnitus: a review. HEARING REHABILITATION QUARTERLY, 1984, 9(2), 9–11.

MEADOW, K.J. and SWIFT, T.R. Tinnitus from intracranial hypertension. NEUROLOGY, 1984, 34, 1258–1261.

MESOLELLA, C. *et al.* Objective tinnitus due to peritubal myoclonus. ORL, 1984, 46, 50–56.

MILLS, R.P. and CHERRY, J.R. Subjective tinnitus in children with otological disorders. INTERNATIONAL JOURNAL OF PEDIATRIC OTORHINOLARYNGOLOGY, 1984, 7, 21–27.

MITCHELL, P.L. *et al.* Computer-aided tinnitus characterization. CLINICAL OTOLARYNGOLOGY, 1984, 9, 35–42.

MOLLER, A.R. Pathophysiology of tinnitus. ANNALS OF OTOLOGY, RHINOLOGY AND LARYNGOLOGY, 1984, 93, 39–44.

ON his tinnitus, LANCET, 1984, 2(8403), 629. (Sonnet.)

OPITZ, H.J. and VON WEDEL, H. On the limited benefit of electrical stimulation in tinnitus suppression. ARCHIVES OF OTO-RHINO-LARYNGOLOGY, 1984, 239, 119. (Summary.)

PANEL 2. Tinnitus and sudden hearing loss. AMERICAN JOURNAL OF OTOLOGY, 1984, 5, 492–493.

PATERSON, J.K. Tinnitus and the cervical spine. JOURNAL OF THE ROYAL SOCIETY OF MEDICINE, 1984, 77, 987. (Letter.)

PENNER, M.J. Equal-loudness contours using subjective tinnitus as the standard. JOURNAL OF SPEECH AND HEARING RESEARCH, 1984, 27, 274–279.

POTTHURST, S. The torment of tinnitus. NURSING MIRROR, 1984, 158(21), 34–36.

PULEC, J.L. Tinnitus: surgical therapy. AMERICAN JOURNAL OF OTOLOGY, 1984, 5, 479–480.

ROTHERA, M.P. Ear disorders: tinnitus. PHYSICIAN, 1984, 2(1), 455, 457–458.

RUBIN, W. Tinnitus evaluations: aids to diagnosis and treatment. JOURNAL OF THE OTO-LARYNGOLOGICAL SOCIETY OF AUSTRALIA, 1984, 5, 201–202.

STEPHENS, S.D.G. Historical origins of the treatment of tinnitus. NEWSLETTER (BRITISH TINNITUS ASSOCIATION), 1984, 26, 16.

STEPHENS, S.D.G. The treatment of tinnitus: a historical perspective. JOURNAL OF LARYNGOLOGY AND OTOLOGY, 1984, 98, 963–972.

SWEETOW, R.W. Cognitive-behavioral modification in tinnitus management. HEARING INSTRUMENTS, 1984, 35(9), 14, 16, 18, 52.

TINNITUS. LANCET, 1984, 1(8376), 543–545.

TINNITUS RESEARCH GROUP, UWIST, CARDIFF. Attempts to produce relief from tinnitus by masking sound. NEWSLETTER (BRITISH TINNITUS ASSOCIATION), 1984, 24, 2–4.

TOLAND, A.D. *et al.* Velo-pharyngo-laryngeal myoclonus: evaluation of objective tinnitus and extrathoracic airway obstruction. LARYNGOSCOPE 1984, 94, 691–695.

TYLER, R.S. and ARMES, D. Conrad- Masking of tinnitus compared to masking of pure tones. JOURNAL OF SPEECH AND HEARING RESEARCH, 1984, 27, 106–111.

TYLER, R.S. *et al.* Postmasking effects of sensorineural tinnitus: a preliminary investigation. JOURNAL OF SPEECH AND HEARING RESEARCH, 1984, 27, 466–.

VALLIS, R.C. and MARTIN, F.W. Extracranial arteriovenous malformation presenting as objective tinnitus. JOURNAL OF LARYNGOLOGY AND OTOLOGY, 1984, 98, 1139–1142.

VON WEDEL, H. and OPITZ, H.J. Long-term therapy of tinnitus with hearing-aids and tinnitus-maskers: a report on three years experience. ARCHIVES OF OTO-RHINO-LARYNGOLOGY, 1984, 239, 119. (Summary.)

AXELSSON, A. and SANDH, A. Tinnitus in noise-induced hearing loss. BRITISH JOURNAL OF AUDIOLOGY, 1985, 19, 271–276.

BIHARI, J. *et al.* Low-powered ultrasound as a treatment for tinnitus: a pilot study. CLINICAL OTOLARYNGOLOGY, 1985, 10, 290. (Abstract.)

BLAYNEY, A.W. A sequential double blind cross-over trial of tocainide hydrochloride in tinnitus. CLINICAL OTOLARYNGOLOGY, 1985, *10*, 97–101. BRIX, R. & EHRENBERGER, K. Auditory brain-stem potentials during slutamic acid and slutamic acid diethylester infusions on patients with tinnitus. ARCHIVES OF OTO-RHINO-LARYNGOLOGY, 1985, *241*, 108. [Abstract.]

CHERMAK, G.D. Continuous and interrupted noise as tinnitus maskers. HEARING INSTRUMENTS, 1985, *36*(8), 10, 12, 14.

COLES, R.R.A. *et al.* Measurement and management of tinnitus. Part II. Management. JOURNAL OF LARYNGOLOGY AND OTOLOGY, 1985, *99*, 1–10.

ENGELBERG, M. and BAUER, W. Transcutaneous electrical stimulation for tinnitus. LARYNGOSCOPE, 1985, *95*, 1167–1173.

GATES, G.A. Management of patients with tinnitus. ARCHIVES OF OTOLARYNGOLOGY, 1985, *111*, 631–632. (Letter in response to R.W. Sweetow, Archives of Otolaryngology, 1985, *111*, 283–284, with reply by R.W. Sweetow.)

HALLAM, R.S. *et al.* A comparison of different methods for assessing the 'intensity' of tinnitus. ACTA OTO-LARYNGOLOGICA, 1985, *99*, 501–508.

HAZELL, J.W.P. *et al.* A clinical study of tinnitus maskers. BRITISH JOURNAL OF AUDIOLOGY, 1985, *19*, 65–146.

HAZELL, J.W.P. Management of tinnitus: discussion paper. JOURNAL OF THE ROYAL SOCIETY OF MEDICINE, 1985, *78*, 56–60.

HULSHOF, J.H. and VERMEIJ, P. The value of carbamazepine in the treatment of tinnitus. ORL, 1985, *47*, 262–266.

HULSHOF, J.H. and VERMEIJ, P. The value of tocainide in the treatment of tinnitus: a double-blind controlled study. ARCHIVES OF OTO-RHINO-LARYNGOLOGY, 1985, *241*, 279–283.

IRELAND, C.E. *et al* An evaluation of relaxation training in the treatment of tinnitus. BEHAVIOUR RESEARCH AND THERAPY, 1985, *23*, 423–430.

ISU, T. *et al.* Paroxysmal tinnitus and nystagmus accompanied by facial spasm. SURGICAL NEUROLOGY, 1985, *23*, 183–186.

JACKSON, P. Electrocochleographic findings and the effects of lidocaine on tinnitus in non-hearing ears. JOURNAL OF LARYNGOLOGY AND OTOLOGY, 1985, *99*, 667–670. JACKSON, P.A comparison of the effects of eighth nerve section with lidocaine on tinnitus. JOURNAL OF LARYNGOLOGY AND OTOLOGY, 1985, *99*, 663–666.

JACKSON, P. Tinnitus and the cervical spine. JOURNAL OF THE ROYAL SOCIETY OF MEDICINE, 1985, *78*, 513. (Letter in reply to Paterson.)

JAKES, S.C. *et al.* A factor analytical study of tinnitus complaint behaviour. AUDIOLOGY, 1985, *24*, 195–206.

LETOWSKI, T.R. and THOMPSON, M.V. Interrupted noise as a tinnitus masker: an annoyance study. EAR AND HEARING, 1985, *6*, 65–70.

MARKS, N.J. *et al.* A controlled trial of hypnotherapy in tinnitus. CLINICAL OTOLARYNGOLOGY, 1985, *10*, 43–46.

MAURIZI, M. *et al.* Contribution to the differentiation of peripheral versus central tinnitus via auditory brain stem response evaluation. AUDIOLOGY, 1985, *24*, 207–216.

MEIKLE, M. and VERNON, J. Tinnitus: a hearing disorder with multiple treatments. HEARING INSTRUMENTS, 1985, *36*(8), 6, 8, 64.

PERUCCA, E. and JACKSON, P. A controlled study of the suppression of tinnitus by lidocaine infusion. JOURNAL OF LARYNGOLOGY AND OTOLOGY, 1985, *99*, 657–661.

REED, H.T. *et al.* Amino-oxyacetic acid as a palliative in tinnitus. ARCHIVES OF OTOLARYNGOLOGY, 1985, *111*, 803–805.

ROUILLARD, R. *et al.* Pulsatile tinnitus: a dehiscent jugular vein. LARYNGOSCOPE, 1985, *95*, 188–189.

SCOTT, B. *et al.* Psychological treatment of tinnitus: an experimental group study. SCANDINAVIAN AUDIOLOGY, 1985, *14*, 223–230.

SHEA, J.J. Medical treatment of tinnitus. ACT OTO-RHINO-LARYNGOLOGICA BELGICA, 1985, *39*, 613–619.

SHELDRAKE, J.B. *et al.* Practical aspects of the instrumental management of tinnitus. BRITISH JOURNAL OF AUDIOLOGY, 1985, *19*, 147–150.

SHULMAN, A. *et al.* Electrical tinnitus control. ACTA OTO-LARYNGOLOGICA, 1985, *99*, 318–325.

STEPHENS, S.D.G. & CORCORAN, A.L. A controlled study of tinnitus masking. BRITISH JOURNAL OF AUDIOLOGY, 1985, *19*, 159–167.

STEPHENS, S.D.G. & HALLAM, R.S. The Crown Crisp Experimental Index in patients complaining of tinnitus. BRITISH JOURNAL OF AUDIOLOGY, 1985, *19*, 151–158.

SURR, R.K. *et al.* Effect of amplification on tinnitus among new hearing aid users. EAR AND HEARING, 1985, *6*, 71–75.

SWEETOW, R. Counselling the patient with tinnitus. ARCHIVES OF OTOLARYNGOLOGY, 1985, *111*, 283–284.

THEDINGER, B. *et al.* Cochlear implant for tinnitus: case reports. ANNALS OF OTOLOGY, RHINOLOGY AND LARYNGOLOGY, 1985, *94*, 10–13.

TINNITUS management: a multi-centre study of patients with tinnitus and their management by masking: BRITISH JOURNAL OF AUDIOLOGY, 1985, *19*, (2).

TREATMENT for tinnitus, DRUGS AND THERAPEUTICS BULLETIN, 1985, *23* (11), 41–43.

VERNON, J.A. Research in tinnitus: a report of progress. ACTA-OTO-RHINO-LARYNGOLOGICA, 1985, *39*, 621–637.

VERNON, J.A. & FENWICK, J.A. Attempts to suppress tinnitus with transcutaneous electrical stimulation. OTOLARYNGOLOGY – HEAD AND NECK SURGERY, 1985, *19*, 385–389.

VERNON, J.A. and FENWICK, J.A. Attempts to suppress tinnitus with transcutaneous electrical stimulation. OTOLARYNGOLOGY – HEAD AND NECK SURGERY, 1985, *93*, 385–389.

WALSH, W.M. and GERLAY, P.P. Thermal biofeedback and the treatment of tinnitus. LARYNGOSCOPE, 1985, *95*, 987–989.

YAMAMOTO, E. *et al*. Tinnitus and/or hearing loss elicited by facial mimetic movement. LARYNGOSCOPE, 1985, *95*, 966–970.

HULSHOF, J.H. and VERMEIJ, P. The value of flunarizine in the treatment of tinnitus. ORL, 1986, *48*, 33–36.

JAKES, S.C. *et al*. Matched and self-reported tinnitus: methods and sources of error. AUDIOLOGY, 1986, *25*, 92–100.

KEMP, S. and PLAISTED, I.D. Tinnitus induced by tones. JOURNAL OF SPEECH AND HEARING RESEARCH, 1986, *29*, 65–70.

YOUNGSON, R. How to cope with tinnitus and hearing loss. London: Sheldon Press, 1986.